YOGA FOR WARRIORS

YOGA ★ for WARRIORS

BASIC TRAINING IN STRENGTH, RESILIENCE
& PEACE OF MIND

BERYL BENDER BIRCH

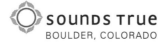

sounds true
BOULDER, COLORADO

Sounds True

Boulder, CO 80306

© 2014 Beryl Bender Birch

Photographs © 2014 Elizabeth Watt

Sounds True is a trademark of Sounds True, Inc.

Published 2014

Cover and book design by Rachael Murray

Cover photo © Robbins Point Photography

Printed in the United States of America

Library of Congress Cataloging-in-Publication Data
Birch, Beryl Bender.
  Yoga for warriors : basic training in strength, resilience, and peace of mind : a
    system for veterans and military service men and women / Beryl Bender Birch.
      pages cm
  Includes bibliographical reference.
  ISBN 978-1-62203-348-5 (alk. paper)
  1. Astanga yoga. 2. Yoga—Therapeutic use. 3. Post-traumatic stress disorder—
    Alternative treatment. 4. Veteran—Mental health. 5. Soldiers—Mental health.
    I. Title.
  RA781.68.B58 2014
  613.7'04608697—dc23
                                              2014011462

Ebook ISBN 978-1-62203-386-7

10 9 8 7 6 5 4 3 2 1

CONTENTS

Warrior Awareness

How Yoga Can Help

Tips on Taking a Yoga Class

Special Tips for Warriors with Physical Limitation
or Disability

Introducing the Warriors Photographed in this Book

Getting Your Attention in Present Time

Body and Mind Together

Mindful Awareness

Gaining Control through Observation

The Source of This Path

Stimulating or Relaxing the Nervous System

The Sound of the Ujjayi Breath

Practicing the Ujjayi Breath

Preparation for Asana Practice

Sun Salutation (Positions 1–9)

Closing Your Sun Salutation Practice

A Healing Flow

FIGURES

This is a book about a yoga practice—*your* yoga practice. It was written primarily for you: military service members—men and women—veterans, warriors, soldiers, sailors, airmen, coast guardsmen, and marines, both active and reserve members of the National Guard and the Reserves, as well as for government workers, contractors, journalists, and anyone deployed to a war zone. I have never been in the military. I have very little idea of what it feels like, as Charles Hoge writes in *Once a Warrior, Always a Warrior,* "to live with danger, convoy in dangerous sectors, be shot at, travel 'outside the wire'," or to live with the constant threat of attack. But I do know what it feels like to do yoga in all its forms—movement, breathing, and meditation. I have been practicing yoga, daily, since 1971, teaching yoga to athletes since 1974, and using yoga practices to help first responders and those with post-traumatic stress (PTS) since 2001.

I was living in New York City at the time of 9/11. Two days after the tragedy, my friend JoAnn Difede, director of the Program for Anxiety and Trauma Stress Studies (PATSS)—called to see if I might be available to help the families of burn victims who escaped from the towers. JoAnn wanted someone with extensive professional experience in yoga to assist the people who were flooding her offices.

As an expert in post-traumatic stress disorder (PTSD), as it—then a very little known condition—was called at the time, JoAnn was at the center of enormous demand to treat the firemen, policemen, city workers, government workers, Con Edison employees, employees of the corporations that had been affected (like Marsh & McClennan and Cantor Fitzgerald), National Guardsmen, and families of those who had perished or were missing—as well as anyone who had escaped from downtown or was working in the post-attack rubble and cacophony. The media called her nonstop for quotes about what people were feeling, network news stations called for interviews, hospitals around the county called looking for advice on treating traumatized Americans. Unexpectedly, JoAnn was the go-to person for expert advice on PTSD.

When I phoned her back, it took awhile to get through. When she finally answered, her voice was rushed as she described what she was facing in her office.

"Isn't there something you could do," she asked., "just to help them sleep or have a moment of relief from their overwhelming grief? Have them breathe or meditate or something? When can you come? Now?"

When I walked into a small room in the hospital burn center, I was nervous. It was filled with comfortable couches and chairs, a plain wooden table, and just a few men and women—relatives of the people who were wrapped in bandages from head to toe and heavily medicated for relief from unbelievable pain. Many were dying, others struggling for life. Their family members sat in stunned silence.

They all looked up as I came into the room, hoping for news of someone, somewhere. They looked exhausted. No one had slept since the towers collapsed. I didn't assume anything. I didn't assume I could help. I didn't assume I knew anything that could be of use. Faced with such incredible suffering, how could anyone go on with the mundane activities of life? There was such a sense of despair in the room. I just sat down quietly at the table and put my head in my hands.

Dear Lord, I thought, *give me strength and the right words to say.* A man came over and put his hand on my shoulder. We both started to cry. That was it—the icebreaker.

I introduced myself and suggested that we, all together, see if there was something we could discover, something we could do, that would help us all to sleep, to deal with the tragedy, to grieve while avoiding despair and depression. I remembered what I had done in yoga classes the night before: sitting with everyone and breathing. It was the breathing that seemed to offer the most relief and the most comfort.

"Let's just sit together," I suggested. Everyone moved into a circle around the table, and I invited them to close their eyes. What happened after that, I don't remember very well, except that I slowly came around to teaching them a closed-mouth yoga breathing technique called *ujjayi.* Breathe in, breathe out—with sound. That's all. You just pay attention to the sound and see if you can make the inhalation and the exhalation the same length and make them sound as much alike as possible.

Within minutes, everyone at the table was making the slow, controlled, aspirant sound of the inhalation and the deep, sibilant sound of the exhalation. They just *got* it. They hung on it as a lifeline. Time became timeless. We sat like that for nearly thirty or forty minutes, although none of us had a clue how long we had been there. I kept an eye on them. Each of them just climbed into the breath and went to a place that was quiet and peaceful—for a moment. One man fell asleep during the session; God bless him. It was joyful to see him sleeping. Another woman actually smiled and came and hugged me. I can't say it was some miraculous cure for suffering, but it did help.

I said to the group, "I hope you will remember that well enough to use in your most difficult moments; it will help you to sleep and to find strength."

The man who had been sleeping looked up and asked, "Can you come back tomorrow?" So I did.

In the long run, the program developed at the burn center was so well received that it became a model for using yoga therapy to manage pain and stress and help with post-traumatic stress. JoAnn's staff of psychologists learned the breathing technique and, in turn, taught it to their patients. Months later, the PATSS received a grant from the Greater New York Hospital Association that funded a program for yoga classes and training in ujjayi breathing for hospital employees. I initially taught the course, and then passed it on to a number of teachers whom I had trained. The program is still growing and bringing much-needed stress relief to employees at Weill Cornell Medical Center.

Thanks to JoAnn's urgent call for help after 9/11, I became one of the first yoga professionals to apply yoga methodology to the integral treatment of post-traumatic stress. As I look back over my twenty-two years of teaching in New York City—with tens of thousands of students in my classes over that time—I'm sure that, unbeknownst to me, many were veterans, and no doubt many were helped by the postures, the breathing, and the meditation techniques we taught.

But it wasn't until after 9/11 that the medical community began to realize just how helpful the broad spectrum of mindful yoga therapies could be for anxiety disorders and post-traumatic stress, when intentionally integrated into more traditional medical forms of treatment such as cognitive behavioral therapy, virtual reality therapy, or eye movement desensitization reintegration (EMDR).

This realization has since spread, and yoga and its mind-body practices are now viable medical treatment alternatives and support systems. Today, extensive research is being conducted—some of it even funded by the Department of Defense (DOD) and the Department of Veterans Affairs

(VA)—that shows how conscious breathing, mindfulness meditation, a practice called *yoga nidra* (or yoga sleep), and the practice of the yoga postures are all—in the case of the DOD study—helping veterans heal and recover from debilitating mental and physical injury.

Thanks to research at places like Harvard University, the Preventive Medicine Research Institute, the Arizona Center for Integrative Medicine, the UMass Memorial Medical Center, the UCLA Mindful Awareness Research Center, and many other prestigious institutions, yoga and meditation now have scientific support as a means for reducing stress, improving attention, boosting the immune system, and promoting a general sense of health and psychological well-being. The scientific community is finally confirming what yogis have known for thousands of years: the mind can heal the body and itself.

When we face a perceived threat—anything that startles or scares us or is stressful or unexpected—our body's reaction is to turn on the fight-or-flight response. This response, which erupts instantaneously in the oldest part of our brain, fires up the stress hormones, cortisol and adrenaline, and gets us ready to either run away from the perceived danger or, if we think we can overpower the threat, to stand our ground and fight. This response is not necessarily a bad thing. The two hormones are a helpful and life-saving part of our body's response to stress and have saved our ass as a species for tens of thousands of years.

But it is important that the opposite reaction, the relaxation response, also be activated when the stress has passed so that the body's functions can return to normal. This means we need to settle down and relax when the high-stress event is over. However, when the body's stress response is activated so often that we don't have a chance to relax, to come down and to return to normal, we end up in a state of chronic stress. Continuous stress, no matter what the source—be it reexperiencing a traumatic event, being deployed for the first time or continuously deployed, or our husband, wife, or boss yelling at us—takes its toll on our lives, our health, and our relationships.

Dr. Herbert Benson, the well-respected Harvard professor and author of *The Relaxation Response,* coined the term *relaxation response* over thirty years ago. He explained it as the polar opposite of the fight-or-flight response. One of the ways in which yoga works is by facilitating the activation of this response. Yoga practices give us things to do that bring our attention into the present moment through focusing on our breath, on our yoga posture, on a gazing point, or through the use of a variety of other yoga tools. In addition to the many physical benefits of a yoga practice that you might already be aware of, such as building strength, flexibility, balance, and agility, the corresponding mental effort to bring mindful attention to the present moment (in a safe and predictable environment like a yoga studio or gym or your living room) unites the body and mind. The effort to focus on the present moment steadies the mind, pulls it back into the body, and can create a calming and balancing response. This brings about many other physical and emotional benefits such as lower blood pressure, slower respiration and heart rate, and calmer, quieter mental activity that can directly contribute, over time, to improvement in overall quality of life—mental, emotional, and physical. That is surely something that can be a welcome aid to a returning veteran struggling to make sense of and adjust to a radically different environment than the one he or she just left. A regular yoga practice, whether meditation, breath work, or moving through postures, can help anyone in the military deal with the stress of facing deployment, being in the field itself, or transitioning back to civilian life.

WARRIOR AWARENESS

Yoga develops awareness, and military training does the same. Almost all the military service men and women, both veterans and active duty, with whom I have worked, seem to be pretty conscious and aware of what is going on around them. That heightened awareness is perhaps what has helped you to survive, to be here now, reading this book. But that hypervigilance can turn into a liability rather than an essential tool for survival, and become a threat to your health and well-being.

In his book, *Once a Warrior, Always a Warrior*, Charles Hoge, a psychiatrist and retired US Army colonel, describes post-traumatic stress (PTS) as a paradox. Unlike "combat stress reaction"—which is an immediate reaction to severe stress on the battlefield, is not a mental disorder, rarely becomes PTS, and is treated immediately with rest and reassurance—PTS is defined by medical professionals as a specific set of symptoms that have gone on for at least a month. These symptoms fall into three categories: avoidance, reexperiencing, and hyperarousal. The irony is that every symptom is an essential survival skill in a war zone and that every one of them can also be a perfectly normal response to life-threatening events.

Everyone experiences trauma in life. Some people experience more catastrophic trauma than others. Not everyone who experiences trauma develops post-traumatic stress. In fact, relatively speaking, very few do. We don't really know all the reasons that some people recover quickly while others struggle with lingering effects all their lives. Clearly there are many determining factors involved—genetics, upbringing, family history, personal health, and others. The fifth edition of the *Diagnostic and Statistical Manual of Mental Disorders* (*DSM-5*), categorizes post-traumatic stress as a trauma and stress-related disorder. But this diagnosis is changing. Post-traumatic stress is *not* an emotional or even a psychological disorder; it is a physiological condition that affects the functioning of every aspect of the body—the skeletal system, the cardiovascular and immune systems, inflammatory response, and hormone system balance. Yoga directly affects the physiological condition of all these various biomechanical and neurobiological systems, which is the main reason that the various yoga practices such as movement, breathing, and meditation can be so helpful. More and more, the preference for dropping the word *disorder* is finding its way into the medical lexicon, and many trauma specialists—both psychologists and psychiatrists—are in agreement that the condition is a *normal* response to an *abnormal* event, and not a psychological *disorder*. For this reason, I have chosen in this book to refer to post-traumatic stress (PTS), as simply that, and not as post-traumatic stress disorder or PTSD.

HOW YOGA CAN HELP

Although warrior awareness can be an asset to help you see danger before others do and be more sensitive and compassionate to others' suffering, the trick is to balance the ability to be aware and maintain the positive aspects of that sensitivity—without allowing that hypervigilance to run amok. Yoga can help. Although it isn't a magic bullet and not intended as a substitute for therapy or as treatment for PTS or any specific disorder, it can help you to ramp the hypervigilance down. It is possible. And you, as a warrior, have great training for this work. You are a natural for yoga. The main difference I see between the discipline of being in the armed forces and the discipline of yoga is that the final objective in military training is to prepare the warrior for battle with an external force or enemy. In yoga training, the preparation is also geared toward battle, but the enemies are within!

If you are wondering how yoga can help you and your family restore a sense of normalcy to your lives after or during deployment, following are a few of the most frequently reported benefits received by the Give Back Yoga Foundation. This nonprofit, which I cofounded, supports yoga programs for military personnel all over the country and gathers feedback from veterans and active duty military members who are regularly practicing mind-body healing techniques like those found in the yoga practices of movement, meditation, and breathing exercises. The list of benefits is pretty amazing, and we continue to hear experiences like these every day:

- reduction of anxiety and depression

- better ability to regulate anger and hypervigilance

- improved concentration

- increased ability to relax

- increased focus on the positive rather than the negative

- greater mental clarity

- pain relief

- more oxygen in body to help repair wounds, burns, and physical injuries

- lower blood pressure

- improved sleep

- increased ability to deal with the mental and emotional strain of combat

- greater access to peace of mind

- support in addiction recovery

Some of the letters and emails we have received from our students and the students of our friends and colleagues tell us many warriors are recognizing the benefits of yoga in helping to manage and process their combat experience and "navigate life after war."

I started yoga when I was in the Marines. It helped calm me down when I was feeling extremely anxious. When I got out, I really needed something to relieve my anxiety, anger, trauma, and depression. Eventually I got tired of feeling so negative about everything and so bad about myself. I had a bunch of injuries, and because I had trouble working out the way I once did, I had a lot of pent up energy in my mind and body. I [eventually] became a yoga teacher, and everything started to change. I learned to meditate, to breathe deeply, and to feel like I had some control of my mind when I felt lousy. Yoga saved my life.

CAPTAIN, US Marine Corps

When I first began yoga in 2001, the vast majority of military members were very doubtful about its benefits. Since then, more and more military personnel are accepting yoga. It is amazing how word spreads, and how much people like it. Military personnel don't realize how much they need yoga until they try it.

US NAVY OFFICER, practicing in Iraq

I am an active duty soldier with over twenty-five years of service in the US Army. I have been jumping out of airplanes for about nineteen of those years. Last year, I went crashing through some trees on an airborne operation and hit the ground harder than normal. I was diagnosed with degenerative disc disease with arthritis. I'm currently deployed to Iraq and have incorporated yoga into my physical fitness regimen. My back feels great without the muscle relaxers and painkillers. Yoga has been the candy for my spine. I will be doing yoga well into my senior citizen years.

SERGEANT MAJOR, US Army

Whether you are just entering military service, preparing for deployment, or returning home after service, the transition from where you are to where you are going can be tough. The journey back home, for example, is a welcome thought but a challenging shift. You are not the same person you were when you deployed. You have changed, and life back home has changed. You have been trained in the skills of a warrior. These skills have served you well and can continue to serve you well. There is no reason to unlearn them. But some of these skills, which are essential to survival in a war zone, may be a bit over the top for a peaceful and relaxing life at home that is radically different from the place you just left. To be happy and to find your way as a warrior in a civilian environment, these skills might need to be adjusted slightly, ramped up or toned down, to adapt to your new home environment.

Yoga, like warrior training, also teaches skillful means. These means are developed through *practice,* much in the same way as military readiness is gained by a warrior, and in yoga that includes movement, breathing exercises, and meditation practices. These practices also build strength, courage, and awareness—again much like your military training. They help you to feel connected to the world in a positive way, give you firm ground to stand on, and show you ways to successfully *navigate* the tricky waters that lie between military life and home.

TIPS ON TAKING A YOGA CLASS

Whether or not you are ready for or even interested in taking a yoga class at a local studio, this book can be an alternative to attending public classes, or it can be preparation for taking a class at a studio. It can also, of course, be an adjunct to any class you may already be taking. However, no matter how experienced a teacher or yoga studio may be with trauma-sensitive yoga, there is always the possibility of many uncomfortable moments or "triggers" for you. How soon you may be ready to explore a class is up to you. It will be different for every person.

Depending on what studio or school of yoga you stumble into and what teacher you get, there can be physical contact between you and the teacher, the class may be very crowded, it may be hot or even overly hot, or instructions can be given in a very authoritarian or militaristic tone by some teachers. Be prepared.

The sequences presented in this book are pretty much my own invention, based on my personal experience both as a practitioner and as teacher working with veterans and military service personnel, so you probably won't be able to find anyone who teaches this identical sequence, unless it is someone I trained. If it is helpful to you, you can find a listing of teachers who have been certified by me on my website, berylbenderbirch.com.

SPECIAL TIPS FOR WARRIORS WITH PHYSICAL LIMITATION OR DISABILITY

This book is for everyone, all warriors, regardless of limitation or disability. One of my students—a young, fit, and very tight veteran with one severely disabled arm—called recently to tell me about a modification he had figured out for an arm balancing posture called Crane Pose. I have always taught that *all* of the yoga practices—from movement to meditation—can be helpful to everyone because each posture and physical movement can be adapted. I asked this student for any tips he could offer warrior brothers and sisters who want to try yoga but

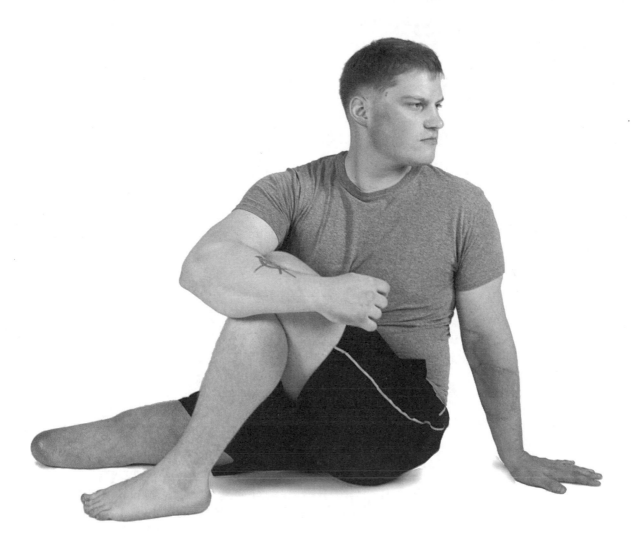

FIGURE I.1 Seated Twist Posture

might feel discouraged from attempting the physical practices due to physical limitation or disability. He said, "Just start where you are and do what you can. That's what I did."

Over the many years I have been teaching yoga, I have worked with a vast assortment of people with many different limitations, injuries, and disabilities. When designing a practice for an individual, with whatever limitation they might experience, I always go back to the basic practice as it is presented in this book and then I work from there. Along with my student, I look at a posture, and together we figure out how we *can do this posture* rather than why we can't do it.

There is always something you can do. Ann Richardson Stevens has been teaching yoga in Virginia Beach military settings for many years. She specializes in adapting yoga for individual needs and works with a number of marines and navy SEALs, both in her studio and at various bases in the area. She shares my can-do approach. For example, one of her students cannot do standing postures because one of her legs was amputated. But the student can do the upper body part of the posture, so she does that.

Do what you can. If you can pick up this book and look through it, you can do this yoga stuff. Approach the book one page at a time. Work your way through it. If there is something that doesn't work for you, for one reason or another, don't just dismiss it. See if you can figure out a way to adapt or modify the posture or practice so that it does work. If you can't do the standing postures, try a variation while seated. If you are lying on your back in a hospital bed and can't move much, then just do the breathing practices. Because the most fundamental and important aspect of nearly every yoga practice is the breath. It is the "secret" key to how yoga works.

Breathing with awareness helps to regulate the nervous system, balance the energetic fields, and heal the body and mind. Plus, everyone can breathe. So breathe. Consciously. Learn the ujjayi breathing technique in chapter 2 and use it in the morning, at night, in the car, at work, or whenever you need physical or emotional balancing. As you approach each posture or breathing exercise or meditation practice, think about the benefits this particular practice might bring you. Then do a little. Do a little more. Be patient. Get a friend to do it with you. It will help. It will change you. You will feel better. And pretty soon, you will find yourself wanting to share these practices with others and become a conqueror who vanquishes enemies—not the enemies "over there," but the enemies within.

If you need help personalizing your practice through modifications, turn to the International Association of Yoga Therapists to find someone local. Or you could find an experienced yoga teacher familiar with teaching yoga movement to persons with physical disabilities by emailing the Give Back Yoga Foundation.

INTRODUCING THE WARRIORS PHOTOGRAPHED IN THIS BOOK

Shane Billings, Sergeant, US Marine Corps. Shane lives in Pennsylvania and is pursuing an undergraduate degree at Penn State University.

Timothy Cole, Specialist, US Army. Tim lives in Crescent City, California, and is attending online college for an associate degree in renewable energy.

Elizabeth Corwin, Lieutenant, US Navy. Liz is a former F/A-18 pilot who lives in Stuttgart, Germany, and can be found upside down on her yoga mat or traveling teaching yoga workshops.

Philip Duguay, Lance Corporal, US Marine Corps. Phil lives in Great Barrington, Massachusetts. He manages a local hardware store, loves to garden, and grows his own food.

Alex Hampton, Lieutenant Commander, US Navy. Alex is currently a F/A-18 pilot and lives in Virginia Beach, Virginia, with his wife and three kids. He has accumulated over 2,500 flying hours and over 400 arrested landings with multiple deployments in Iraq and Afghanistan.

John R. Morgan Jr., Specialist 4, US Army, and Sergeant, Connecticut National Guard. John lives in Griswold,

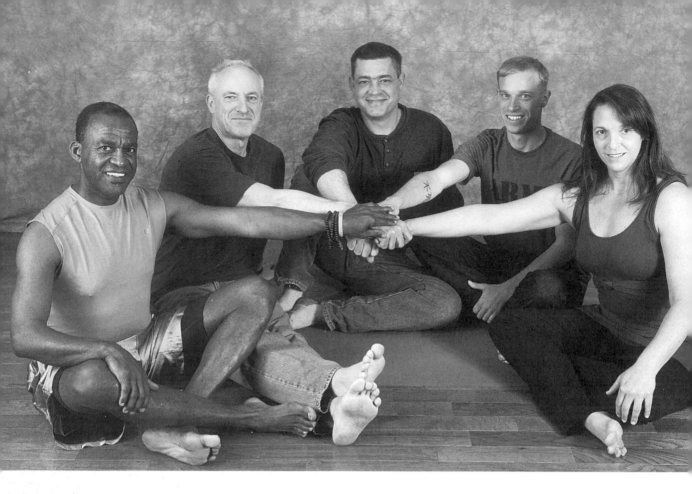

FIGURE I.2 Thanks to Our Warrior Yoga Models.
From left: Mike, John, Phil, Tim, Melinda.

Connecticut. He owns a petroleum contracting company and enjoys farming and pottery.

Melinda Morgan, Lieutenant Colonel, US Air Force. Melinda lives in Virginia and is a public affairs officer with multiple deployments, most recently to Afghanistan for one year. She loves to paint and cook.

Michael A. Riley, Sergeant, US Air Force. Mike, a self-employed courier, lives in Bloomfield, Connecticut. He finds peace of mind through his yoga practice and now teaches yoga.

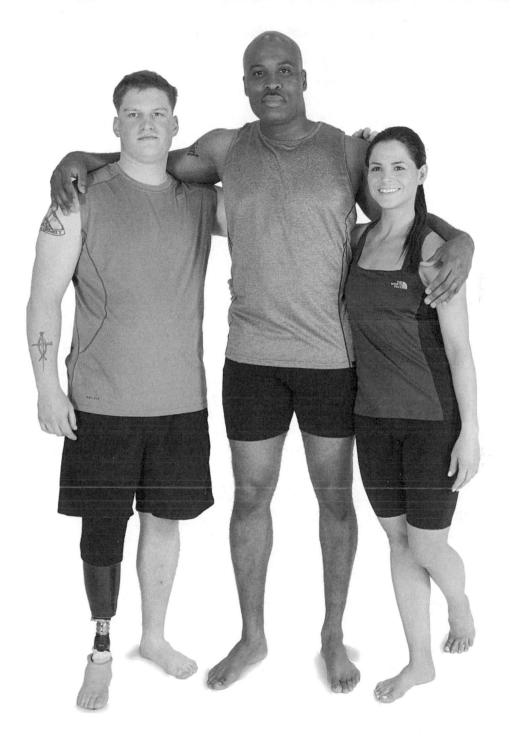

FIGURE I.3 Thanks to Our Warrior Yoga Models.
From left: Shane, Alex, and Liz.

CHAPTER 1

THE PEACEFUL WARRIOR

Something happens to people who practice yoga regularly. They change. They may not have planned to change, other than maybe becoming a little more flexible or healing an injury, but they do change. And not in a way they expected. In the forty-plus years I have been teaching, I have asked thousands of people with a regular practice the following question: "How many of you feel that yoga has changed your life?" Everyone *always* raises a hand. There has never been one person who hasn't. Now really, that isn't so remarkable. Everything changes all the time; you don't need to do yoga to experience change. That's true. But then I add, "I assume it was for the better." They laugh and say, "Yes, for the better."

So here are all these people saying that yoga has changed them and that the change has *improved* their lives. Now that is a little unusual. It isn't random change. As a long-time yoga practitioner, I can say with some degree of certainty that this is a different kind of a change—it isn't exactly a conscious change because it sneaks up on you.

But it is a directed change. You take up yoga, in any of its many forms—whether the physical practice of the postures *(asanas)* or the breathing practices or mindfulness meditation—and then you practice regularly without a break and with some kind of personal involvement of your heart. This means you commit to it, you are earnest in your discipline to show up and just do it. You don't have to talk about it. You don't have to share it. You just have to do it. And lo and behold, change starts to happen. Transformation!

GETTING YOUR ATTENTION IN PRESENT TIME

How does that change happen? Well, yoga—in all its forms and expressions—teaches you to center, to pay attention. Yoga is about focusing on one thing, and then working to keep that focus on that one thing without distraction or interruption. That's the training. Whatever you are doing, whatever the point of focus—maybe it is the breath, maybe a prayer or word, or maybe a yoga posture—the work is about making the effort to hold the focus on that single point. When you learn to pay attention, to hold focus on the present moment, you *slow down.* Not in a sleepy, lazy, passive sort of way, but in an alert, clear, relaxed sort of way: heart rate, breathing, mind activity, muscle tension all slow down and relax. Your body gets a break from the tension your mind generates. You feel better. You are better. In that moment, you are creating life and longevity for yourself. You are more relaxed. And guess what: you are actually more content, and eventually, more *happy.*

This book is about helping you learn how to focus on one thing, which will in turn, get your attention into present time. I understand that the present moment, at times, can be hell. Why in the world would we want to be here? "Here" sucks at times.

The advantage is that as you train yourself to be present and stick with your practice come hell or high water, there is less and less room in your head for the noise about the past and the future; consequently, the stressful effects on your body are reduced. The present moment is where life is truly lived and is the only place it is truly lived. Think about it. What's the option?

Whenever we aren't "here," where are we? Well, our bodies are always here. We can't get around that. But our minds . . . oh, our minds, where are they? They can be anywhere: disconnected from our bodies and drifting around; off on their own as if they had no connection to us at all; stuck in the past or frightened of the future; reexperiencing old traumas or dreading new experiences; and causing us all kinds of havoc—anxiety, indigestion, sleeplessness, irritableness, panic attacks, and a host of other conditions and illnesses that we really don't need to list here.

But the truth is that, even when our minds seem to be off on their own and not "here," they really *are* here. All the internal dialogue that goes on when we have been injured, traumatized, insulted, ignored, or disrespected, and all the drama, the turmoil, the internal conversations, the reexperiencing, the fear of the next moment doesn't happen out in space somewhere. It happens in the body. The body hears it, responds to it, absorbs it, and believes it. Our cells do their best to carry out their responsibilities and maintain our health and wellness, but it must get a little discouraging for them at times, when the mind is constantly in a state of distress and broadcasting negative and fearful energy. No wonder we have indigestion or can't sleep.

BODY AND MIND TOGETHER

The body and mind are inextricably connected, even though a good bit of the time they seem to be in different worlds.

To heal from trauma or injury means to get our body and mind working together on the same page, supporting one another and giving each other positive reinforcement. That is what happens when we start practicing yoga. The word *yoga* means "union." It refers to the link between the body and mind, and it strengthens our awareness of the impossibility for either one of them to exist independently. As a result of yoga practice, we start to notice little changes. We have moments of feeling whole. Our internal dialogue shifts just a smidgeon. The conversations we have with ourselves in our head—that dialogue that seems to go on endlessly—quiets a little bit. You know the conversations I mean: the two different players, arguing back and forth about the "right" course of action. They never stop talking! If we had a spouse or a roommate like that, what would we do? Throw them out. And yet here is that endless noise in our very own mind going on and on and on. In yoga, we are able to diffuse this a bit and quiet it down. We become a little less critical of ourselves and a little more tolerant, more supportive and gracious to ourselves. We see a light at the end of the tunnel. And that inspires us to continue our practices, as they seem to be working. We have a moment of being grateful, happy even. Maybe we *can* get better, improve our outlook, direct our lives the way we want them to go, and as we continue, the light gets brighter.

MINDFUL AWARENESS

As I explained in the introduction, the awareness that the yoga practitioner works to cultivate is not all that different from the gripping concentration and focus required of a soldier doing maneuvers in a combat zone—a raw and penetrating step-by-step sensitivity to what energy is surrounding the moment and what is potentially incoming. Learning to pay attention in a beneficial way is at the very core of yoga practice. It means simply to get your attention in present time, to work on keeping the mind steady, to be mindfully aware of what is going on moment to moment.

But unlike the life-saving and necessary hypervigilant awareness of moving about in a war zone, where the awareness is directed outward and continuously scanning the external world, in yoga practice, it is just the opposite. The awareness is directed inward. To master yoga to the same degree of efficiency as keen military readiness, the only thing a highly trained warrior needs to do is *change the direction of focus*—from out to in.

Doing this involves focusing our awareness on the movement of the breath and feeling sensations in the body as they are arising. Developing mindful awareness through yoga simply means working to be present, observing what is going on within ourselves at any given moment. It takes practice and study, just like developing marksmanship. But perseverance pays off. The mind begins to slow down. We start to notice and accept what comes up, just as it is. So, instead of squirming around because we are feeling uncomfortable with the thought or memory of something painful, we just stop, and look, and feel whatever it is that is making us uncomfortable. Maybe it is tightness in the stomach, tightness in the chest, shortness of breath, or sweaty hands. There is something physical that is accompanying the stressful thought. The clue is there; we just have to notice. As soon as we notice what the physiological response is, we can take a breath and consciously relax, or reach out and take control of ourselves to ramp the response down. Instead of stuffing the feeling down and mentally maneuvering things around to make ourselves more comfortable, we stop and acknowledge whatever *it* is—in this moment. We notice and accept what *is* in this moment. That's the first step.

GAINING CONTROL THROUGH OBSERVATION

Accepting what is in the present moment means that our focus is directed, for example, at the movement of the breath, and our attention is aimed at *observing,* or *witnessing,* our experiences, thoughts, and feelings as they arise. We are no longer *identified* with thought; we are the *observers* of thought. This is a really important distinction, and once it is actually experienced, the difference becomes quite clear. See if you can feel this.

When your mind is jumping around like a monkey, that becomes *who you are* in that moment. You feel like you are being thrown around, like a paper cup floating in the sea. You're up, you're down, you're depressed, you're elated, you're here, you're there. The noise is unbearable. But when you take a step back and observe the process, instead of being *in it,* you can disconnect from the monkey mind and just *watch* the acrobatic display. You become an observer. You realize that you are not your thoughts! You can say, "Oh look, here I am, getting stressed, getting panicked, having this thought, having that thought. Wow, look at how busy my mind is. Going at warp speed. Instead of getting swept along, I can step aside and *choose* to take another path. Let me just take a breath and focus on how that feels." This can liberate you from feeling trapped, as if you had no choice about what you're feeling or experiencing. You now feel in control.

This is a big shift, and putting this new way of operating into effect can take something like a leap of faith—trusting that this methodology is going to work for you and really will help you to overcome the effects of trauma and/or anxiety. As you begin to practice the exercises in this book and experience some of their benefits, your understanding of how this all works will deepen, and it will become easier to keep up with the practices. The actual experience of yoga can't be described or defined because it is an experience, and as such, has to be *experienced!* All you have to do to begin reaping the benefits is follow the instructions. The closest we can come to actually talking about the result of practice is to say that it is an unequivocal sense of connectedness, of regaining wholeness and peace of mind. Yoga provides us with a logical, and even scientific, system for going deep within—beyond the information delivered by our five senses—to find the source of our being, to find stillness and joy, and to find answers to some of our most profound questions.

THE SOURCE OF THIS PATH

The specific practices offered in this book are from a two-thousand-year-old traditional form of yoga referred to as Classical, or *Astanga yoga* in Sanskrit (the original language of yoga). The word *astanga* comes from the two root words, *ashto* (eight) and *anga* (limb). These eight limbs delineate a brilliant methodology that can take us to a deep and clear understanding of who we truly are. They start us out on the ground floor, offering a solid foundation and anchoring us to the earth like the roots of a grand and wise old tree. And as we grow and become more rooted, we are safely able to climb from limb to limb, going higher and seeing farther. I know this sounds a little woo-woo, but once you get going with the practices, you will understand what I mean.

The first five limbs *(yama, niyama, asana, pranayama, pratyahara)* are considered the *outer* limbs and, relatively speaking, are the easiest to follow. Except for the first limb, which is a set of five ethical principles that are called the *yamas* and serve as a foundation for a dedicated yoga practice, the remaining four outer limbs all have to do with stuff you can actually do with your body, such as move (asana) and breathe (pranayama), and are relatively tangible. The yamas, or restraints, are traditionally called the *great vows* because they are timeless and universal and apply to all people, at all times, regardless of nationality, religion, heritage, or race. They tell us not to steal, lie, be violent or greedy, and not to wear ourselves out by chasing every skirt or pair of pants that passes our way! These five yamas are meant to set us on a trajectory of conscious behavior. They are meant to point us in the right direction and should be kept in mind as we move into our yoga practices. We do the best we can in our adherence to the yamas, and the longer we go on practicing, the greater our understanding of these ethical considerations becomes. For example, not stealing comes to mean not only not taking some material object that doesn't belong to us, but also not taking time or energy or ideas that don't belong to us, whether taken from another person, another being, or even from our home, Mother Earth. This expands the yamas into becoming a deep form of ecology and reverence for our environment.

The second limb is called *niyama*, which means "observance," and there are five of these as well. They include suggestions like: be content, be clean, exercise and do something every day that burns out impurities, study with wise teachers, and get your attention in present time. Not a bad list. Unlike the yamas, these are a little more practical and are, for the most part, simple things we can do as part of our daily routine.

In this book, much of our preparatory work will be with the third and fourth limbs, which are asana (the practice of the postures) and pranayama (the practice of yogic breathing). *Asana*, the third limb, literally means "seat" and refers to the yoga postures or movements. The whole point of doing the yoga postures, or asanas, is first to get us into our bodies; and then to rejuvenate, heal, cleanse the body, ground and center us physically and mentally, calm and quiet the mind, and prepare us for deeper yoga work, like conscious breathing and meditation. These postures can be challenging as well as a lot of fun to do, a good workout, and a great way to start the day.

Pranayama, the fourth limb, comes from the word *prana* meaning "energy," comparable to the word *chi* in the martial arts. Since the word yama means "control" or "restraint," we can think of pranayama as "energy management" or "energy control." Literally, pranayama refers to a variety of yogic breathing techniques. But the pranayama practices are a way of training ourselves to pay attention to what we are doing with our energy. What are we giving our attention to? We learn to focus on our breath and learn to notice what distracts us. This helps us to be more aware of things we do or think about that might be draining us, exhausting us, or even making us sick!

According to yoga philosophy, our efforts in the five outer limbs prepare us for the more subtle practices of the last three limbs, the *inner* limbs, of concentration, meditation, and realization, and which we will move into in chapters 8 and 9. Sometimes the fifth limb, *pratyahara*, which means an "inward turning of the senses," is thought of as the bridge between the inner and outer limbs. You will see in chapter 8, when we begin work with the practice of *yoga nidra*, or "yoga sleep," how this technique starts to turn our attention inward to a place of deeper focus.

The inner work picks up where the outer work ends. We leave behind the world of the body and move into working with only the mind. Although this is a silly distinction, since the body and mind are impossible to separate, in the inner world of meditation, we no longer work with physical movement or conscious control of the breathing. It's just directing the mind onto a point of focus that is more subtle than our previous work. The practice of meditation, which is really the primary point and practice of these last three branches on our yoga tree, relies on the previous training in concentration and focus that we did in asana and pranayama in order to find the awareness and stillness, both mentally and physically, that is necessary to move into this deeper work. Asana is historically regarded in yoga as just practice for meditation. It is like preparing to run a marathon. We need to practice the shorter distances, like the 5K and 10K, before we can attempt the longer distance.

There are many different schools and styles of yoga—many of which can be helpful for a variety of disorders, illnesses, and injuries. Some are gentle, some are hot, some are vigorous, some are simple, some complicated. There are almost as many schools and approaches as there are people looking for classes. The practices in this book are a middle path. They are simultaneously hard and soft, active and restorative, and yes, at times will be difficult but will also become easier! Once you start practicing, you can begin to make choices for yourself as to what works and what you need to do to find balance and wellness. Yoga, in all its forms—asana, breathing, meditation—is a therapeutic system and can be healing and helpful for all of the conditions mentioned previously, as well as many others. Yoga therapy isn't just something you seek out if you are ill or injured. The therapeutic element should be integral to your practice. Your practice should help you heal from trauma and injury, and even, perhaps, help you in the coming years to avoid pain, illness, arthritis, or unnecessary surgery.

As I mentioned in the preface, today there is greater cooperation between traditional, Western medicine and alternative systems of healing from around the world. The combined knowledge of the best of Western and Eastern traditions has come to be known as *integrative medicine*. More and more, people are finding that their friends, families, and physicians are recommending they start yoga. For those of us who have been practicing and studying for decades, it is encouraging to see that yoga has begun to be accepted by the medical world as a legitimate aid to stress management, wellness, and healing.

CHAPTER 2

EXPAND INTO VICTORY

BASIC BREATH WORK

There is a powerful yoga breathing technique that is an incredibly effective way to get grounded, get present, get control, and ramp down almost instantly. It is called *ujjayi pranayama,* and you can easily learn to do it anytime, anywhere. The word *ujjayi* means to "stretch or expand" (*uj*) into "victory" (*jayi*)! Very cool. Ujjayi pranayama means "victorious breath" and is a closed-mouth breathing technique that will be the supportive pillar and primary tool of the asana practice that we will begin in the next chapter. But to make it easier to learn, we are going to focus on this powerful breathing technique first, as a stand-alone practice that is portable, powerful, and an extremely important tool to have in our toolbox of mindfulness techniques.

Ujjayi breathing does two important things. First, it serves as a way to help us pay attention. The breath itself creates a distinctive sound at the back of the throat. The purpose of generating a sound is to give us something to listen to. Consciously creating this audible whishing sound works to hold our focus in the present moment. We focus on the breath, we listen to the breath, and we control the breath. It is a good feeling. To do the ujjayi breath, you have to pay attention. It doesn't just happen like your natural breath. For example, while you are sitting and reading this page, you are breathing, but you probably aren't aware of your breathing. But with ujjayi breathing, you create the breath. It is a conscious breathing technique that only happens when you are aware that you are doing it.

The second thing that ujjayi breathing does is create heat, helping to turn on the sweating mechanism. This isn't the most important thing when you use this breath on its own as a tool for relaxation or ramping down, or a way to "take a beat" before you slam someone over the head who's walked up behind you and startled you. But it *is* important to the practice of the yoga postures. If you come from an athletic background, plus basic training and possibly several years of deployment, you probably feel as if your body is made of steel and will never bend. That's why this breathing technique is so important. When you are moving and focusing and using this breath, it gets you warmed up and sweating, which makes the whole practice of the postures so much more doable. So, getting the body hot and pliable is essential. Even iron will bend if you heat it up.

When used to support our asana practice, the exhalation portion of ujjayi breathing becomes subtly but consciously linked to letting go, or releasing, and the inhalation portion to standing firm. Both are used to fuel the fire, or the *agni*. This breathing technique, as you will experience for yourself when we begin to tie it into the movement in the next chapter, creates tremendous heat in the body, and through this stoking of the fire, you will be able to *burn* toxins in both your body and mind!

You may wonder why we use a closed-mouth breathing technique in our yoga asana practice. You might be used to lifting weights, for example, and are in the habit of huffing or blowing out through the mouth as you lift. When mouth breathing, as we do when we are running, for example, we inhale and exhale air quickly and in large volumes. This is fine for any kind of aerobic activity. Hyperventilation, or the release of too much carbon dioxide too quickly, as can happen when we repeatedly exhale forcefully through the mouth, can cause arteries and blood vessels to constrict, not allowing the oxygen in our blood to reach our cells in sufficient quantity. But when we run, since we are producing more carbon dioxide as a result of a major increase in activity, our forceful out-breathing isn't an issue because it is important that we *do* breathe out more CO_2 in order to maintain the proper oxygen/carbon dioxide balance in our blood. Conversely, in yoga, we aren't creating as much carbon dioxide, so it isn't necessary to breathe out through the mouth. Doing so can also throw us out of chemical balance. Lack of sufficient oxygen going to the neurons of the brain can activate the sympathetic nervous system, which, in turn, accelerates the heart and triggers the fight-or-flight response, making us feel tense and irritable. When we consciously breathe only though our nose, we are apt to breathe more deeply and engage the parasympathetic nervous system, which slows the heart rate and relaxes and calms the body.

STIMULATING OR RELAXING THE NERVOUS SYSTEM

The *sympathetic* and *parasympathetic* nervous systems are like the "wake me up" and "slow me down" divisions of the autonomic nervous system (ANS), which is the motor division of our general nervous system that regulates organs and other functions such as heart rate, digestion, muscle tension, brain wave activity, skin temperature, and natural respiration. For most systems in the body, the sympathetic portion amps up activity, and the parasympathetic portion quiets things down. Years ago, we called this part of our nervous system the "involuntary" nervous system—meaning that we really didn't have any control over things like heart rate and muscle tension and brain wave activity. But we realize now that it is possible to have a great deal of control over these functions. Things like biofeedback training and yoga practices have taught us that people *can* consciously learn to control aspects of the autonomic nervous system such as heart rate, brain wave activity, muscle tension, blood flow, blood pressure, and skin temperature.

We can get a sense of how these two oppositional aspects of the ANS work through something as simple as taking a breath. When we are startled or surprised, what do we do? We gasp—we breathe in! An inhalation signals the sympathetic nervous system and, for most of the systems in the body, pumps us up—very imperceptibly of course, but it does activate what in yoga is called the solar, or the *pingala,* energy current in the body. When we want to relax or calm down, what do we do? We sigh—we breathe out. An exhalation signals the parasympathetic nervous system, which quiets or relaxes most of the systems in our body—again very subtly— and sends an impulse to the lunar, or *ida,* energy current in our body. According to yoga philosophy, these currents move along tracks in the energy field that surrounds our physical body, and are constantly shifting dominance to maintain balance between arousal and rest. They attune not only to our inner world and needs, but also to the demands and conditions of our environment.

The conscious closed-mouth technique of ujjayi is a powerful means of practicing mindfulness and an excellent practice for ramping down the nervous system when we need to take it down a notch. In conjunction with movement, as we will see in the next chapter, or as a stand-alone practice for stress management (as we are about to practice here), ujjayi breathing can help you break the cycle of anxiety in your life.

THE SOUND OF THE UJJAYI BREATH

Ujjayi is a technique in which you make a sound somewhere between that of the wind or the sea and the sound of Darth Vader. The sound and the breath itself are made through the regulation of the glottis, which is not really a structure or muscle, but the space between the vocal cords. When the muscles that control the vocal cords are adducted, or drawn together, they vibrate as breath is forced over them, creating speech. When these muscles are abducted, or pulled apart, they open the glottis, which allows deep, rapid breathing. The ujjayi sound is formed by partially closing the glottis, forming only a small opening at the back of the vocal cords. This is the same action that creates whispered speech. This reduction in the volume of air passing through the vocal cords creates an increase in the velocity of the moving air and produces the recognizable ujjayi sound.

If you open your mouth and whisper the sound "ahhh," you will notice that you feel a slight contraction at the back and base of your throat as the glottis narrows. Do it again. Notice the sound. Now try to do it on an inhalation, keeping the sound with your mouth open. It's a little more difficult and may make you cough at first. Try it again, a few times—mouth open, "ahhh" sound, in and out.

Now close your mouth and do it again, keeping that same contracted feeling and keeping the sound. Can you feel where the throat (the space between the vocal cords) tightens when you do that, the place way at the back of the palate (way down the throat) where you feel the hiss of the whisper? Inhale and exhale with your mouth closed, keeping the air passing over and through that same spot. If you lose the sound, open your mouth and whisper an "ahhh" again to recapture the feeling. The inhalation is a little more breathy, more *whishy* sounding. The exhalation is a little richer, a little more throaty sounding.

PRACTICING THE UJJAYI BREATH

To help focus your attention just on learning this breathing pattern, either lie down with your head supported on a small pillow or sit cross-legged on a blanket or mat. If you are going to sit, it will be more comfortable if your hips are higher than your knees, so you might want to put a firm pillow or meditation cushion under your butt to elevate your hips. Get comfortable and start to settle into stillness. Once you have arranged your sitting position and no longer feel the need to adjust or fiddle with your seat, close your eyes and start to simply observe the flow of your natural breath, in and out. Do this for two to three minutes. Just watch your natural breath. Don't change it or alter it—just watch.

Now, begin to bring out the ujjayi sound. At first, you may want to just focus on making the sound during the exhalation, as it is a little easier. After you have practiced this for a few minutes, see if you can extend the breath slightly on the exhalation. Here are some additional tips to apply when practicing ujjayi breathing:

- Keep the breathing relaxed and flowing— do not hold the breath between inhales and exhales nor between exhales and inhales.

- Keep your shoulders relaxed.

- Keep the belly relaxed so that as you inhale, you feel the little muscles between the ribs (the *external intercostal muscles*) pulling the ribs apart and expanding the entire chest; and as you exhale, you feel the opposite action, the *internal intercostal muscles* pulling the ribs back in and contracting the chest and thoracic cavity.

- Be gentle and careful not to use too much force as the breath should be strong but not strained, and the sound should be loud enough to be heard by someone sitting next to you but not by someone who is across the room.

Start with a two-minute practice session. Over time, and as you become more familiar with the technique, gradually increase your sessions to five minutes. When this time has passed, gently and slowly return to normal breathing for a minute or two.

If it is physically possible, and if you are in a place where you feel safe and comfortable, quietly lie down on the floor on your back and rest. If you want to, close your eyes. Let your arms rest next to you, slightly out from the sides of your body with the palms face up, and your legs separated about as far apart as your hips, with your feet falling out to the sides. Stay in that position for a few minutes and rest, keeping your eyes closed.

When combined with asana, ujjayi pranayama is the powerful engine that drives and carries a beautiful, flowing, uninterrupted practice. In the next chapter, as you move through the sequence of postures, you will be harmonizing your movement with this conscious yogic breathing technique. As I mentioned previously, when used to support our asana practice, the outbreath helps us to let go and release tension and tightness, the in-breath helps us to be resolute and stand firm. We learn to bring these two opposing forces that are present in every aspect of the universe—expansion and contraction—into balance within ourselves.

CHAPTER 3

BUILD THE FIRE

SUN SALUTATIONS

Yoga had its origins in India, and as in most ancient and indigenous cultures, the sun held a central place in the life and thought of that early civilization. For thousands of years, the day began—all over the planet—with the worship of the sun. Many of our ancestors in ancient cultures such as the Mayans, Incas, Aztecs, Native Americans, Eskimos, Druids, Romans, Greeks, and most likely dozens of others, had sun temples and sun deities. The sun was the symbol of the great light that the human soul longed to find—whether consciously or not—within. Just think about the importance of the sun in our own culture. For starters, without it, we wouldn't be here. The sun gives life to everything we know, we have, we eat, we breathe.

So it is no surprise that a short sequence of movements called the sun salutation (*surya namaskar* in Sanskrit, which translates to "reverence to the sun") is the way most yoga asana methods begin their practice. There really isn't a better way to start. The sun salutation does a really good job of warming up the body for a strong asana practice. It serves as a foundation for the subsequent postures, and is just about a complete workout in itself, as it loosens and heats up every joint and corner of the body.

The sun salutations can be modified to accommodate almost anything—a broken leg, a torn rotator cuff, osteoarthritis in a hip, an amputated limb, a hip or knee replacement, a variety of shoulder injuries, sprained or broken ankles, back injuries, or confinement to a wheelchair. They have been used by people of all ages, by all types of athletes, and by people with all kinds of limitations and restrictions. We just tune in to what we are able to do, and then develop a modified program that will work for us. The great thing is that, without exception, everyone can do the breathing! And once we begin to breathe and move and pay attention to what we are doing, the mind begins to quiet, and the symptoms of anxiety, panic attacks, depression, or PTS will begin to subside little by little.

PREPARATION FOR ASANA PRACTICE

The ways we prepare for and enter our yoga practice can determine how powerfully it works for us. Here are several things to keep in mind as you enter the practice.

Eating

To prepare for the practice of the yoga postures presented in this book, it is best not to eat anything, or at the very most, a light snack like toast or an apple or banana, for at least three hours before beginning.

Hydrating

It is also important to be well hydrated going into the practice. Try to drink at least sixteen to twenty-four ounces of water thirty minutes before practice, and then again after practice to rehydrate your body. Unless you forget to drink plenty of water before you start your practice, you don't really want to drink water or other liquids during practice. Remember, you are trying to build a fire, and what happens when you pour water on a fire? It goes out! Drink beforehand and keep the fire burning while you practice.

Clothing

For ease of movement, wear comfortable workout clothing designed for yoga practice. Nothing too tight but nothing too baggy either, as it will get in your way and possibly be more revealing than you would like.

Flooring

It is ideal to practice barefoot on a clean wood, tile, cement, or bamboo floor using a nonslip yoga mat or just on the floor itself. Do not use anything that will slide around (like a towel or blanket) for a mat, unless you need something under your spine for some of the floor work. In that case, put the towel or small, flat cotton rug on top of the nonslip mat.

Cleanliness

The body and clothes should be clean. You might notice in the first four to six weeks of your asana practice that there may be some unusually strong, strange odors emanating from your body. The asanas are squeezing out toxins and tension (some very old and deeply rooted) and cleansing the cells and organs in ways that sports activities often don't. But after you have been practicing for a month or so, and if you are following a fairly clean and healthy diet, you will notice that your sweat no longer has much of an odor. The whole process of doing asana is about purification, so you want to be clean, pure, and without odor, especially if you are in a class situation. Remember "clean" has no odor, so slathering yourself with synthetically scented lotions, potions, deodorants, soaps, and shampoos is not the same thing and can make others in class sick. No scented anything—just clean!

Distraction

If you are practicing on your own at home, pick a space where you are least likely to be distracted or dismayed. The more neutral the space, the more likely you will be able to feel content with the moment and attentive to the activities of your inner being. Distractions are part of life, and whether they are internal or external, as you learn to focus and direct your attention in your practice, they will bother you less and become less attractive. Eventually, you will be able to let the interfering thought pass and won't be drawn in by external sight or sound. But sometimes a distraction is just too big to ignore. If you become distracted or interrupted, and it is guaranteed that you will many times, *simply notice that you have been distracted.* This is the critical moment. This is when you take hold of your attention, let go of the thought or the distraction, and pull your attention back to your breath. Every time you are able to do this, you become stronger in your resolve to stay grounded and present, and you become healthier and less susceptible to being distracted by sounds, sensations, or painful (or pleasant) memories.

Room Temperature

No air conditioning—being cool may be *cool* but as far as temperature goes, it defeats the whole purpose of the practice. If you don't like sweating, this yoga may not be for you. If you can't sweat for medical reasons, then work easy and breathe easy.

Sweating

Hopefully, by the time you finish doing the repetitions, you will have broken into a sweat. That's the idea. The particular system of asana practice described in this book is what is called a form of *tapas,* or detoxification. The word *tapas* means "to burn." The idea is that you use the work to start an internal fire, which then burns impurities and clears toxins—both physiological and psychological—from the body through squeezing, sweating, and breathing.

Generally, we associate sweating with huffing and puffing and working hard. In yoga, we learn to work hard, but also to work smart. The breath is even, powerful, and controlled, not panting. The heart rate is even and steady, not pounding. We are statically contracting muscles and focusing on those contractions; remember, although you will be stretching, this isn't a stretch class. As we move into postures and hold those positions, we are consciously contracting the muscles opposing the stretch. This will make sense once you start to practice. Those strong, conscious, *static* contractions that happen in stillness are different from the *dynamic* contractions of moving a limb through a range of motion, like lifting or running or biking. The static contractions, along with the ujjayi breathing, help to keep the sweating mechanism turned on and wring the toxins out of the muscles, ligaments, and tendons, as well as out of the brain!

SUN SALUTATION (POSITIONS 1–9)

The sun salutation we are going to work with here is a sequence of nine positions, and each position or movement flows from one to the next. It is performed, once learned, as a fluid sort of dance, with one breath accompanying each move, and is generally repeated several times. The idea is to use this work to warm up for the rest of your practice.

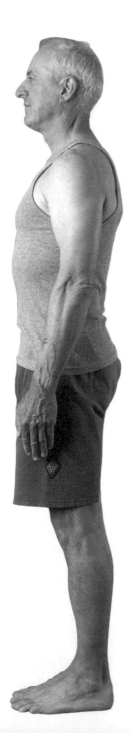

FIGURE 3.1

Mountain Posture

Mountain Posture

Stand at the front of your yoga mat with your feet together and with your arms at your sides. (If that is not possible for reasons of balance or discomfort, then make sure your feet are at least parallel. Press your feet into the earth and feel the earth supporting you. Imagine you can feel energy coming up from the earth through your feet, all the way up through your hips, shoulders, and out the top of your head. Mother Earth—here, now—has your back. It's a good feeling. Make it a good feeling. Level your pelvis, by dropping your tailbone. Pull your belly in, tighten your thigh muscles, and lift your chest bone (the sternum). Take a moment to focus your eyes on a point in front of you: pick a little spot and look at it. Try to hold this gazing point for a moment or two. Begin the ujjayi breathing. Take a moment to settle in and actually *be there*.

This is mountain posture, or it could be called attention position. (See figure 3.1.) You will begin and end your practice in this position and frequently return to it between most of the standing postures for the entire standing sequence.

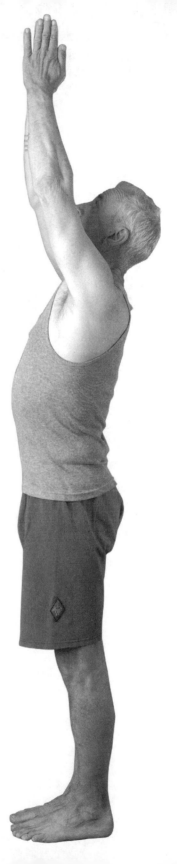

FIGURE 3.2
Sun Salutation,
Position 1

Position 1 **Mountain Posture with Arms Up**

Inhale and raise your arms up over your head, placing the palms together (if possible). Look up. Lift the knee caps by tightening or flexing the thighs (quadriceps). Reach up as strongly as possible, lengthening the torso and lifting the rib cage. Don't arch the back or lean back.

Note: If you have neck issues or it feels painful to look up, then look straight ahead. Stand straight up and down. Keep your belly pulled in and your tailbone lowered. When *contracting,* or *tightening,* your thigh muscle, be careful not to hyperextend the knees; you can soften the knees slightly and still contract the thighs. This lifting of the quadriceps is what I explained earlier as a *static contraction*—a tightening of a muscle without an accompanying movement in the associated limb. A static contraction is the "hard" or tightened aspect of the posture. It takes energy and requires fuel to accomplish. Thus it creates heat. Static contractions are an extremely important element of the practice and are a key component of generating heat, keeping the fire going, and keeping the sweating mechanism turned on during the practice. This procedure of static contraction will be referred to frequently throughout the book.

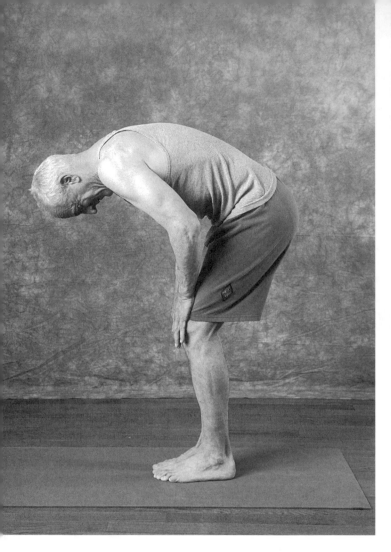

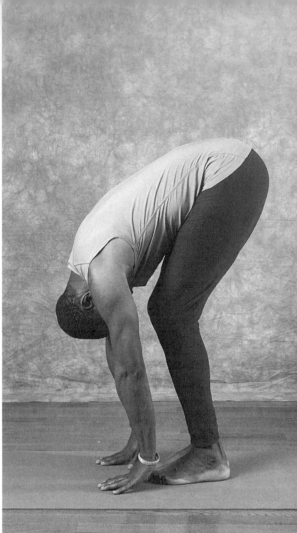

FIGURE 3.3 Sun Salutation, Position 2

FIGURE 3.4 Sun Salutation, Position 2, Advanced

Position 2 **Standing Forward Bending Posture**

Exhale, bend forward, bend your knees, and place your hands on your knees (see figure 3.3 or 3.4). Tuck your nose into your knees. If you are really flexible, you can take your hands all the way to the floor for this position. (See the following note as well as figure 3.4.)

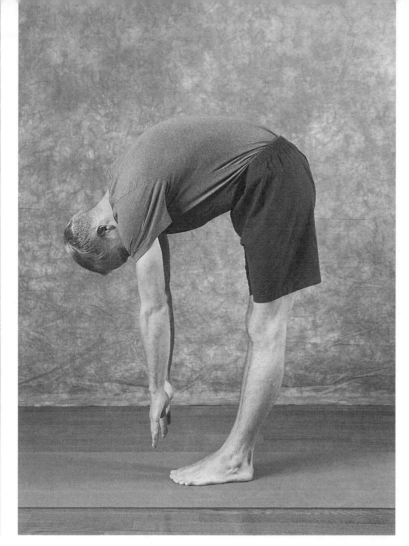

Note: In figure 3.5, it is easy to see in the model, who is a runner and has very tight hamstrings, how stressful standing forward bending can be on the lower and middle back. If you look like this when you bend over, and cannot easily touch your toes, then it is critically important that you bend your knees and place your hands on your knees and not try to reach the floor.

FIGURE 3.5 Sun Salutation, Position 2, Incorrect

Note: Before taking this posture, consider whether you have tight hamstrings, lower-back pain, or any kind of low-back injury. If you do, it is really important to bend your knees as you bend over and that you do *not* try and take your hands all the way to the floor. Standing forward bends attempted with straight legs can be contraindicated and dangerous if the hamstrings are very tight and/or there are lower back issues!

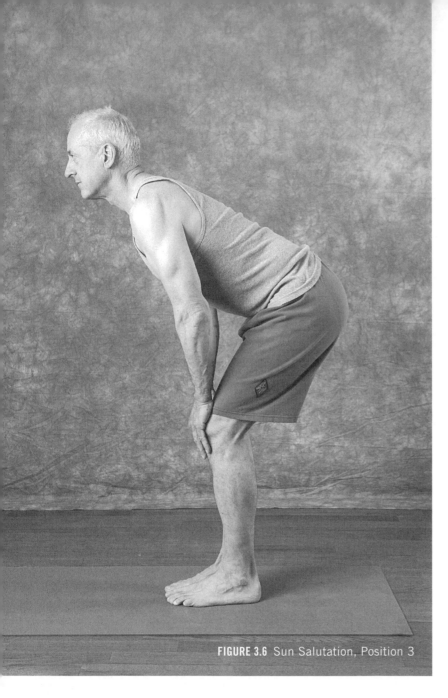

Position 3
Standing Forward Bending Posture, Head Up

Inhale, lift your chest, extend your spine, and look up, keeping your hands on your knees (or the floor).

FIGURE 3.6 Sun Salutation, Position 3

Position 4
Four Limb Stick Posture

Exhale, place your hands on the floor (bending the knees as needed to do so) on either side of your feet, step all the way back, and come into a straight or plank position. (If your hands are already on the floor, just step back to the plank position.)

Inhale again, and then exhale and lower your torso into a push-up position (figure 3.8), hovering above the floor, if possible. (If not, just lower yourself all the way to the floor or just lower your knees, as in figure 3.9, slowly building arm strength over the weeks of practice).

Note: Keep your torso steel-straight and your elbows tucked into your sides. Keep your shoulders level with your butt and your elbows. Don't let your butt sag, but don't stick it up in the air either. Think *plank.* If you are strong enough to hold a push-up without sagging in your hips, then you can do this with straight legs; but if you are not, you can modify this posture by lowering your knees to the floor. Keep your head in line with your spine. Gaze straight in front of you.

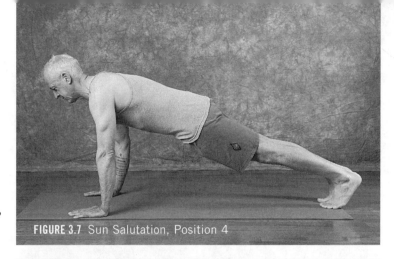

FIGURE 3.7 Sun Salutation, Position 4

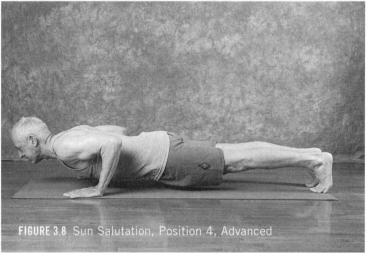

FIGURE 3.8 Sun Salutation, Position 4, Advanced

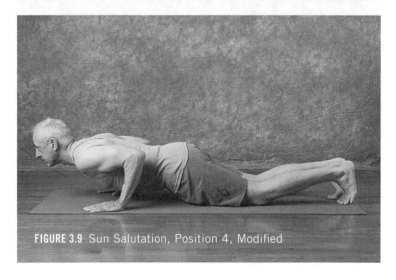

FIGURE 3.9 Sun Salutation, Position 4, Modified

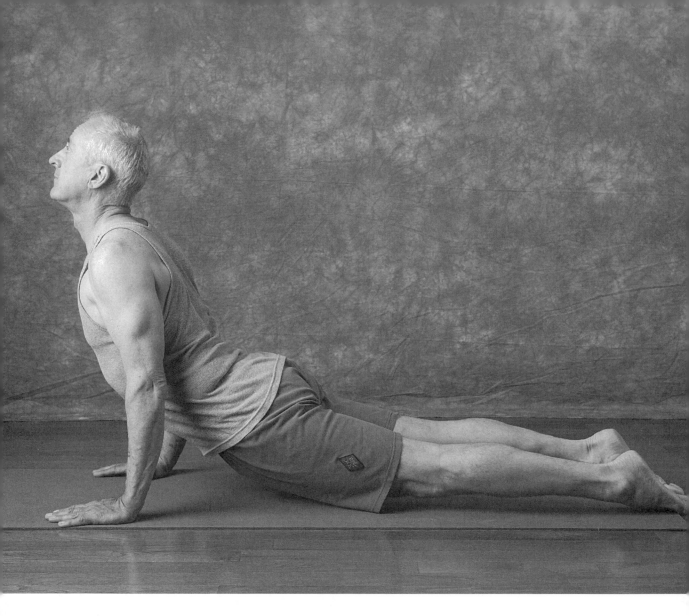

FIGURE 3.10 Sun Salutation, Position 5

Position 5 **Upward Facing Dog Posture**

Inhale; turn the feet so the toes are pointed (plantar flex-ion) and the tops of your feet are on the floor. Lift the body all the way up onto the hands and the tops of the feet only, straightening the arms and rolling the shoulders back. Don't "hang" between your shoulders. Use your deltoids (shoulder muscles)! Look up.

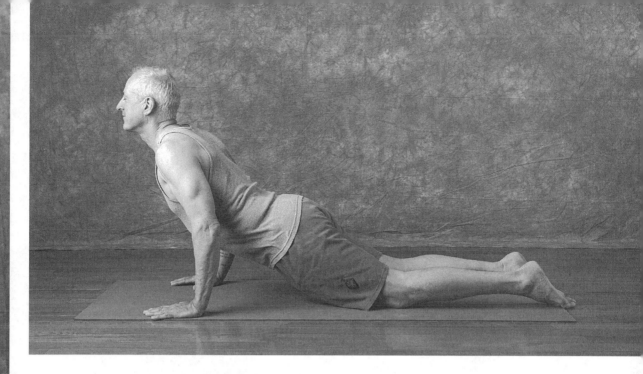

Note: If you have lower-back pain or injury, it is best to use the knees-down modification of this posture, or skip it altogether. If you have limited plantar flexion (find it difficult to point your toes), both versions of this position might be a little uncomfortable, so continue with the knees-down posture until the tops of your feet stretch out a little.

Note: This position can be extremely difficult for a person with tight feet or ankles. It can also create lower back distress if done *incorrectly*. Do not let your back sag or your shoulders hunch up around your ears. When done correctly, this should not be uncomfortable. If you feel too much pressure in your lower back or on the tops of your feet, then modify the posture slightly by placing your knees on the floor, as in figure 3.11.

FIGURE 3.11 Sun Salutation, Position 5, Modified

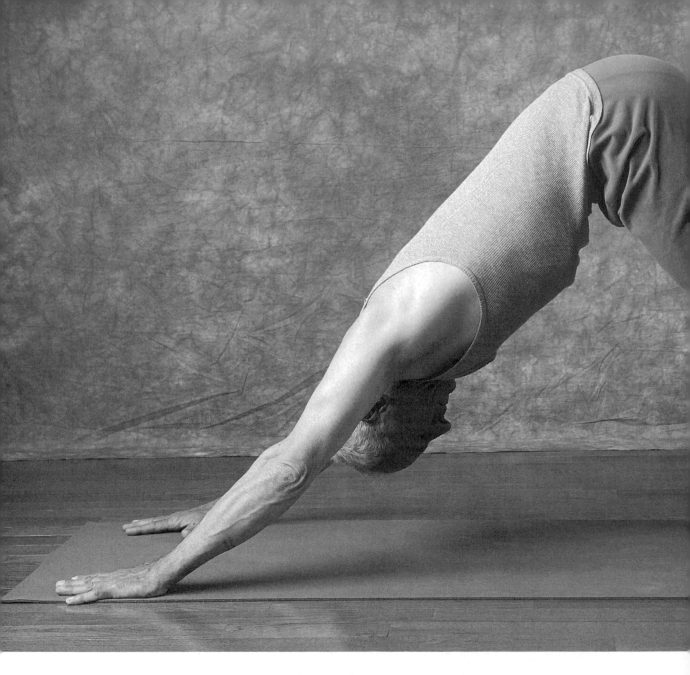

Position 6 **Downward Facing Dog Posture**

Exhale and turn your toes back under (dorsiflex position) with the balls of your feet on the floor. Push up and back into an upside-down V position. Look back between your legs at a point behind you. Let your neck relax and head

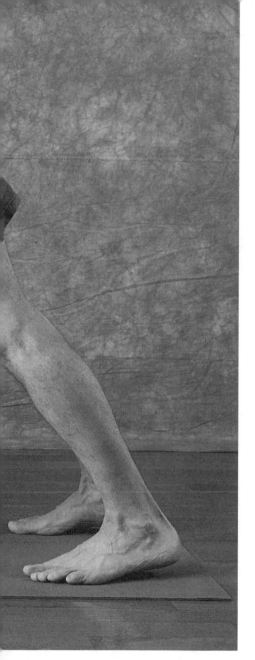

FIGURE 3.12 Sun Salutation, Position 6

Note: Downward facing dog posture (position 6) is an awesome place to hang out. It stretches the hamstrings, the calves, the back, the tendons in your ankles and feet, and strengthens the arms and shoulders. It is an excellent posture for the lower back.

hang, then tuck your chin slightly toward your chest. Push down on your heels. Pull up on the belly. Your arms should be straight, but be mindful not to let your elbows lock (or hyperextend, which means to press inward). From the front, your arms should look very, very slightly like parentheses ( ), with the elbows slightly wider than the wrists and in line with the shoulders, or just wider than the shoulders. The exact details will depend on your personal physiology.

Hold this posture for five complete controlled ujjayi breaths. (A complete breath equals one inhalation and one exhalation.)

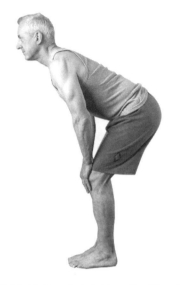

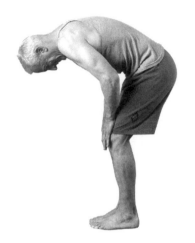

FIGURE 3.13 Sun Salutation, Position 7   **FIGURE 3.14** Sun Salutation, Position 8

Note: If you hop or jump forward from position 6 to position 7, make sure you don't jump into a squat—it's hard on the knees! Just bend the knees as much as necessary to land softly.

Position 7 Standing Forward Bend Posture, Head Up

This is the same posture as position 3, which you did on the way down to the floor.

Inhale as you walk or hop your feet back to your hands. Bend your knees slightly and place your hands on your knees (or the floor, if you can) and extend your spine. Lift the head and look up.

Position 8 Standing Forward Bend Posture

This is the same posture as position 2, which you did on the way down.

Exhale as you round your back slightly and tuck your nose toward your chest, keeping your hands on your knees (or on the floor, if you can). Look down.

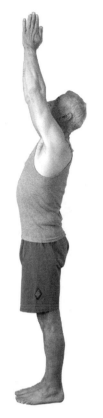

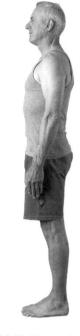

FIGURE 3.15 Sun Salutation, Position 9

FIGURE 3.16 Mountain Posture

Position 9 **Mountain Posture with Arms Up**

This is the same as position 1.

Inhale as you come all the way back to standing straight, arms parallel over your head or palms touching. Reach up. Look up at your thumbs or look straight out in front of you. Remember to hold your belly in, level the pelvis, and lengthen the tailbone down.

Return to Mountain Posture
(Attention Position)

Exhale and lower your arms back down to your sides.

Note: Finish here for a moment, standing with your feet together, spine straight—natural curves in place. Continue to breathe, being aware of the breath. Make sure your belly is pulled in, your pelvis is level, your thighs are engaged (or contracted, which pulls up the kneecaps), and visualize your shoulder blades melting down your back. Keep your gaze steady. Listen to your breath. Keep it even and controlled. Anchor yourself to the earth. Feel supported and connected to the earth.

Repeat

This completes one sun salutation. When you first start your practice, repeat the entire sequence three times. As you become stronger, slowly work up to between five and ten repetitions each session. Once you learn the postures and movements, each salutation will take a little over a minute, about seventy to seventy-five seconds—so you can't say you don't have the time for them. Just learn them and do them and love them.

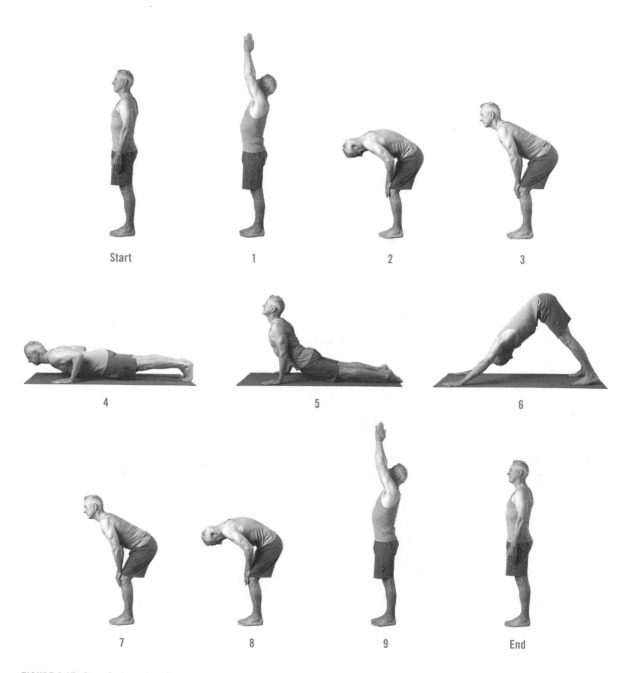

FIGURE 3.17 Sun Salutation Flow

Start　　　1　　　2　　　3

4　　　5　　　6

7　　　8　　　9　　　End

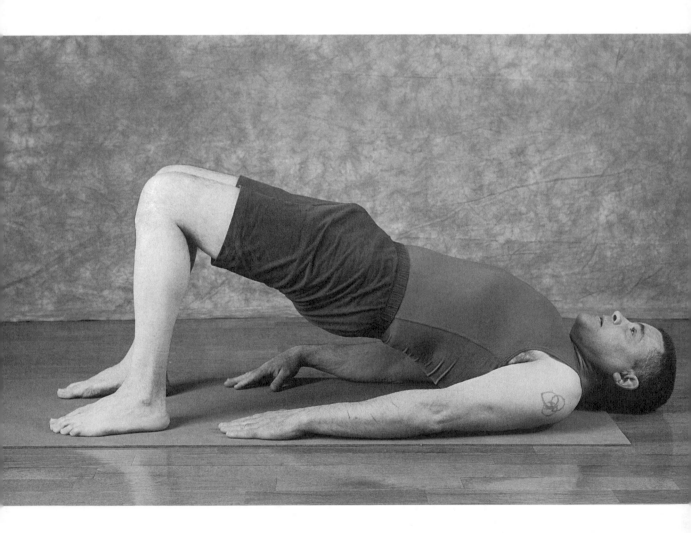

FIGURE 3.18 Bridge Posture

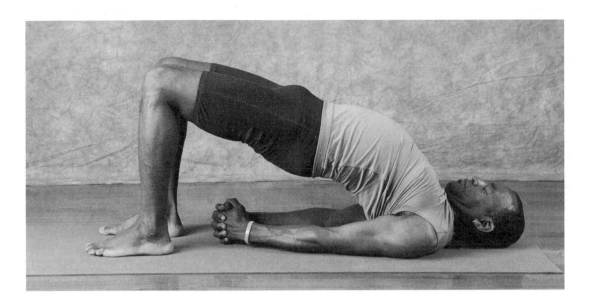

FIGURE 3.19 Bridge Posture, Advanced

CLOSING YOUR SUN SALUTATION PRACTICE

After you have completed your practice of the sun salutations, the following few postures will provide both a slight strengthening and stretching effect for the muscles in the lower back. This should make it possible for you to lie comfortably still in relaxation posture and for the lower back to be relaxed and at ease. If your lower back tends to bother you in general and is still a little cranky after going through this routine, spend a couple more minutes in the knees to chest posture and then return to relaxation posture.

Bridge Posture Lie down on your mat, on your back, and bend your knees. Bring your knees to your chest, then put your feet down flat on the floor in line with your buttock bones. Press your hips up into the air with your arms alongside, palms face down. Take a few breaths here.

Note: If you want to move a little deeper into the posture and stretch out the pecs (the front of your shoulders, *pectoralis major*), bend your elbows slightly and see if you can clasp your hands together underneath your torso. Squeeze your shoulder blades together and see if you can straighten your arms. Eventually you will have all your weight on your shoulders, upper arms, and the back of your head, and your spine will not be touching the floor.

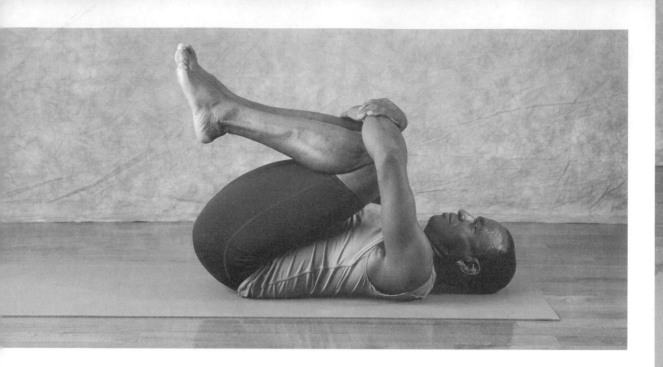

FIGURE 3.20 Supine Knees
to Chest Posture

Supine Knees to Chest Posture Release your hands and lower your hips to the floor, then bring your knees to your chest. Wrap your arms around your shins and give yourself a hug. Then release your arms, but keep your knees pulled to your chest.

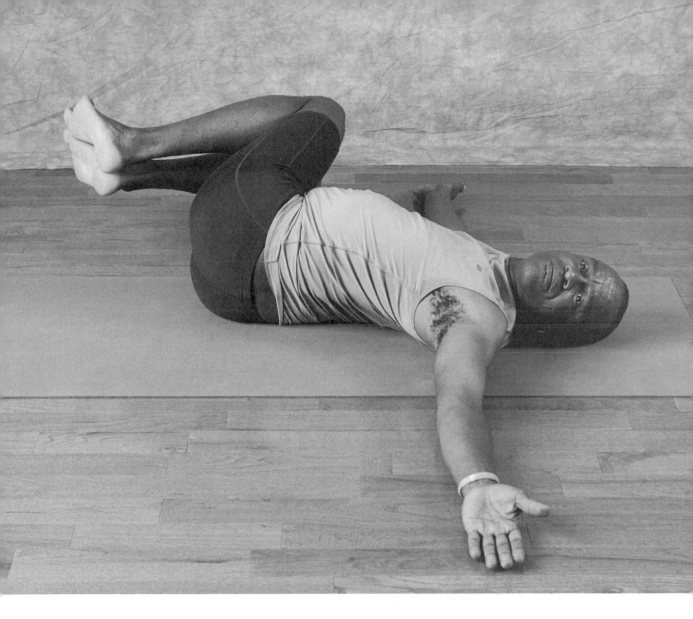

Supine Knees to Chest Twist Posture Reach your arms out to your sides in a T position and roll your knees to your right side, keeping the knees up high toward the elbows. Take a few breaths here, then bring the knees back to center and roll them to your left side. Take a few breaths here as well. Keep your shoulders on the ground as best you can.

FIGURE 3.21 Supine Knees to Chest Twist Posture

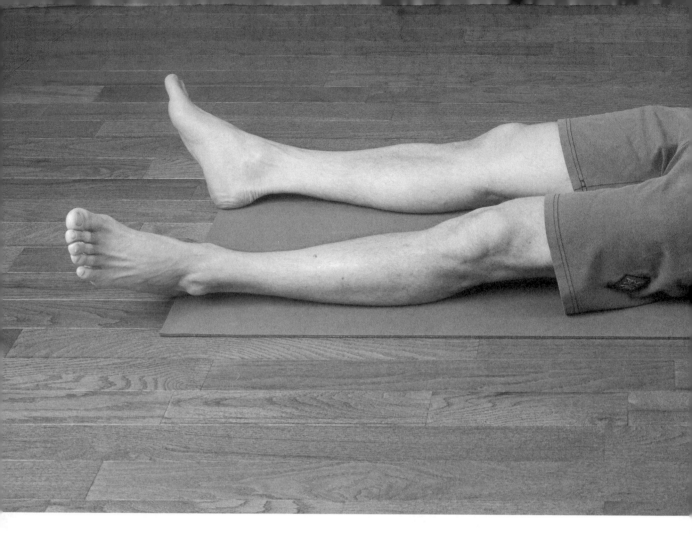

FIGURE 3.22 Relaxation Posture

Relaxation Posture Return your knees to center and stretch your legs out full-length along your mat. Take your feet at least as far apart as the width of your hips, and then let your feet relax and fall open to the sides. Place your arms slightly out from the sides of your body, palms face up, head level. Close your eyes.

If you have chronic lower-back soreness or tightness, this practice should help to loosen the tight muscles and help to heal any injuries or alleviate misalignment. However, if you experience any tightness or discomfort in your lower back when you come into relaxation posture, it may be helpful to place a fairly sturdy pillow, bolster, or folded-up blanket under your knees (see figure 3.22).

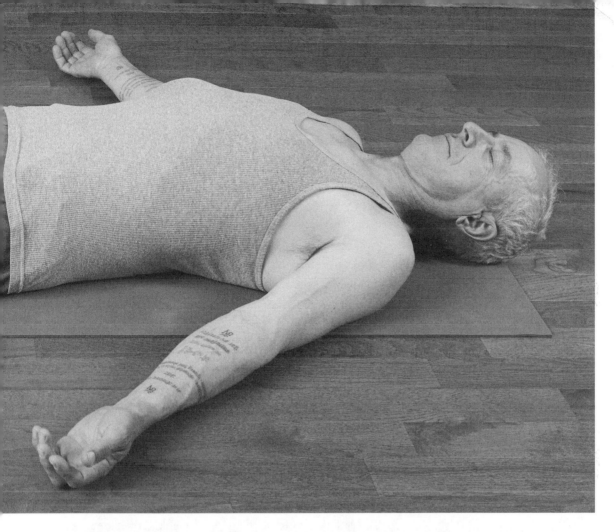

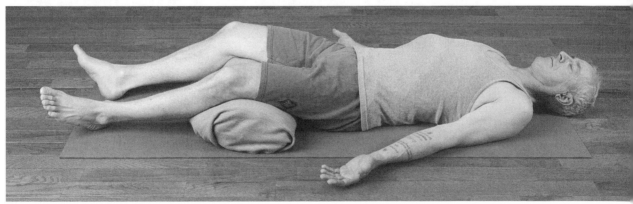

FIGURE 3.23 Relaxation Posture, Modified

See if you can keep your attention on your breathing. Let the breath become quieter and quieter, softer and softer, slower and slower, eventually relinquishing all control of the breath and returning to natural breathing. Stay here as you cool down and drop into relaxation—for at least ten minutes and preferably a few more. You might become so relaxed and your arousal levels may be calmed to such a degree that you actually fall asleep. Good for you! Rest easy. This is an opportunity to have an experience of feeling completely relaxed and at ease, and one that you will come to realize you can duplicate again and again.

A HEALING FLOW

Important reminder: if your back (or any other part of your body) didn't hurt before you began your yoga practice, it shouldn't hurt after your yoga practice. If it does, you are doing something wrong. Go back and carefully read the notes and precautions and work easily until you build strength and endurance in your yoga posture practice and can flow through the postures without creating pain or tension.

As you become more familiar and comfortable with the sun salutations and the idea of linking your movement with your breathing, you will find you are able to glide through this sequence without stopping or putting in extra breaths. You will simply *flow* from one posture to the next, effortlessly, and then from one sun salutation to the next. Practice the sun salutations until you become comfortable with the movement and the breathing.

Do this practice four or five days a week. Let it become second nature. Just do this much to start. Don't rush through this to get on to what's next—it will all come to you in time. Part of your work, remember, is to be present and content with *what is*. It took awhile for you to build the tightness and stress levels, and it will take awhile to ease them out. Once you have practiced the sun salutations for a few weeks, you should be able to move on to the standing postures in the next chapter.

And one more thing: you might want to congratulate yourself for making the commitment to take the step to actually do this. You are consciously choosing to do something to help yourself either feel or be better. This is a huge step. The moment we take effective action to do things that make us feel better, we are already on the road to healing and recovery.

CHAPTER 4

DEVELOP POWER AND BALANCE

STANDING POSTURES

As you build your practice, don't rush through this stuff. Make sure you get it right first. When I said, "Just do this much to start" at the end of the last chapter, I didn't mean just do this much on the first day. I meant for a while—maybe a week, maybe a month. Even if all you ever do is the sun salutations, you will experience some benefit. When you feel ready, move on to the practices in the following chapter. Of course, you can read the next chapter, and in fact, you can read the whole book, but the *practice itself* will take time to develop. If you are in a hurry, yoga is not for you. This practice will not take you from tense to relaxed, tight to flexible, fat to fit, or injured to repaired in twenty-one days or less.

Always keep in mind you are developing a living, ongoing, ever deepening, transformational practice. *This is a discipline.* As a military service person and highly trained warrior, you understand what that entails better than most.

Because yoga is designed to be a discipline, it is a little different from other forms of exercise. In yoga, the word for practice is *abhyasa,* which means "to make an effort to keep your mind steady and focused." Pay attention to whatever it is you are doing—that's what is meant by *practice* in yoga— and if you aren't making that effort, for example, while you are doing asana, then it isn't really practice, it's just exercise. There's nothing wrong with exercise—it just isn't yoga.

This is the big secret, really. This is how yoga works. By uniting your mind with your body, yoga is training your brain in riveting focus. and this is how it can help you begin to recover from depression, insomnia, PTS, and other stress and anxiety related disorders. If you practice, the practice teaches you how to *get your attention into the present moment.* If you are "here," you can't be anywhere else.

Wolfgang Pauli was a professor of theoretical physics at Princeton University, and one of the founding fathers of quantum mechanics. In 1945, he won the Nobel Prize for his exclusion principle, now known as the Pauli principle, which states that no two electrons can occupy the same quantum state. If we think of "here" as one electron and "there" as another electron, it follows that they can't both be in the same place. If your mind is focused on "here," you can't be worrying or reexperiencing "there" (the past). This means that you can begin to exert some control over where your mind is and what effect that "place" is having on your body. We begin to see that we can not be churning our brain and belly, anxious about what might happen tomorrow and truly be mentally and wholly "here" at the same time.

PRACTICE IS LIFE-CHANGING

But suppose you *are* worrying about or reexperiencing the past, and can't shake it. What then? The practice will help you become an objective observer of the experience. "Hey, my body is freaking out here." "My mind is raging." "An emotion is taking me for a wild ride." What happens then? We *notice* we aren't "here"—that we aren't in the present moment—and we plow directly into the tension with our yoga discipline. We drop our awareness into our bodies and tune right into those physiological responses that accompany rising anxiety: the tense belly, the shallow breathing, the sweaty palms, the tightness in the throat, or the pounding of our hearts. Then we go to our yoga tools: the breath; a conscious, deep exhalation; one sun salutation or twenty; a mindful moment of positive self-talk. Eventually, with practice, this can help take you over that hurdle of mental paralysis in which you feel like nothing will ever change or ever get better, and you can't seem to break out of the behavior rut you find yourself in. The effect of practice does help you to move, to inch forward, to begin to feel better.

Because *practice* is defined as "effort toward steadiness of mind," then yoga practice isn't just about asana, or something you do when you are on your yoga mat; it is something that can be done 24/7. Yoga teaches us that if we can learn to pay attention and be present while we are doing sun salutations, then maybe we can learn to pay attention and be present while we are taking a shower, walking the dog, talking with our boss, applying for a job, and standing in line at the supermarket. This is the work, the mindful effort—that moment we catch ourselves and take a breath. This simple act of vigilance is the profound technique that turns on the relaxation response. This is what helps us to sleep at night and gradually shut off the babble of the mind.

PREPARATION FOR THE STANDING POSTURES

This chapter will introduce you to *standing asanas*. There are ten postures in this section of the practice. If you are just starting out, these postures should be learned one at a time, adding maybe one or two to your practice every couple of days. If you have been practicing yoga for some time and are knowledgeable about alignment, then you can integrate the sequence at a somewhat faster pace.

Breathing

Learn the ujjayi breathing. Without it, you simply aren't doing this particular method of yoga correctly. So spend time learning it and practicing it—and not just when you are doing asana, but all the time. It is an incredible tool that you can carry around with you and use anytime you need to chill or take it down a notch.

Don't hold your breath; keep it flowing. Many people who begin yoga practice for relaxation purposes unconsciously hold their breath. As you go along, at least half of your effort is going to be in keeping the breathing "pump" going strongly—not through straining, but through clear focus. Remember, balance between hard and soft.

You will generally be moving up and down into the postures; every movement is accompanied by an inhalation or an exhalation. Listen to the breath and practice paying attention to it. Try to coordinate the duration of a connecting movement with the duration of the breath. Generally, you will be exhaling going into a posture and inhaling coming out.

Once learned, all the postures are meant to be done sequentially, flowing from one posture to the next, from one side to the other, using the breath to move the body in and out of the postures. Many of us feel separated from the world and out of sync! Yoga helps us to feel connected to ourselves and to other people and things around us as well, as a result of learning to link our breathing to our movement.

Playing Music

I'm not an advocate of playing music during practice, as it means you are listening to the music instead of your breath, and it can be distracting and take you off into la-la land. But if it helps you to get started and create a rhythm to your practice, by all means, use music for as long as necessary to get you going.

Posture

Pay attention to the correct alignment of the posture and let your intelligence be stronger than your ego. All the postures require strength, which means some muscles are working! As a warrior, you will more likely be focused on your strength. That's excellent. But don't strain or force a posture. Pay attention to your head and neck—don't let them hang in the postures. The head is an extension of the spine and should be held in alignment with the spine in all the postures. (See figure 4.1, triangle posture.)

Once you have "found" your posture, settle in and try not to fidget. See if you can come to stillness as you take five ujjayi breaths. Keep your gaze steady as well.

Feet

Balance your weight evenly on both feet for all the standing postures. Pay attention to the alignment of your feet. If the directions say turn the right foot out ninety degrees, make sure it's ninety degrees and not eighty-nine. It makes a difference.

Balance of Hard and Soft

Be aware of the balance between the "hard" energy of the muscles that are contracting in any posture and the "soft" energy of the muscles that are relaxed or stretching. Often you will find that you are a bit over the balance point into one end of the spectrum or the other. Too much contraction results in straining, can lead to injury, and often accompanies the practice of someone who feels tense and keyed up all the time. Too much relaxation results in "sleeping" and can lead to not much of anything in terms of change or transformation. This often accompanies the practice of someone who is completely disconnected from the body and avoiding contact for fear of reexperiencing a previous pain, disappointment, or trauma. Find the balance. Get to know yourself.

Pain When Doing Asanas

Remember! If it hurts, you're doin' it wrong! Back off whatever you are doing and modify the posture until it stops hurting. Or skip it altogether.

THE STANDING POSTURES

After you have completed your last sun salutation (as described in chapter 3) and stepped back to the top of your mat, you will begin the first standing posture.

Posture One Triangle

Note: In this posture, consciously holding the quadriceps (thigh muscles) in static contraction on the forward leg is vitally important to the correct practice of the posture. This helps to maintain heat, support the torso, hold the knee in correct alignment, and protect the hamstring muscles at the back of the thigh.

1. Inhale and, from the top of your mat, turn to your right so you are going the long way on your mat. Step your feet about three feet apart. Make your feet parallel, then turn your right foot *out* ninety degrees and your left foot *in* forty-five degrees. The heel of the right foot lines up with the heel of the left foot. Lift your arms so that they are parallel to the floor. Contract the right thigh muscle, lifting the kneecap. If you have a tendency toward hypermobility (your joints easily move beyond normal range), soften or microbend your knee.

2. Exhale, turn slightly to your right, dropping your right hip back slightly, and then bend as far as you can to your right, taking hold of your shin or ankle or whatever you can reach without straining. Extend your left arm straight up toward the ceiling. Turn your head and look up at your left hand. Keep the head in line with the spine—don't let it hang. Keep your arms and shoulders aligned in a vertical plane as best you can. Hold for five breaths.

3. Inhale, come up out of the posture, and reverse your feet precisely.

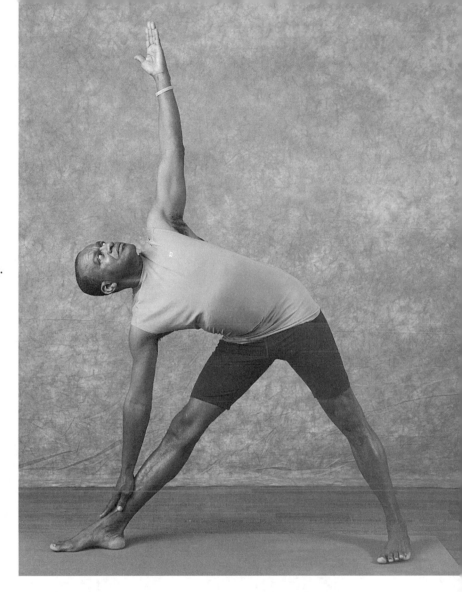

FIGURE 4.1 Triangle Posture

4. Exhale; descend into the posture on the other side. Look up at your right hand. Hold for five breaths.

5. Inhale; rise up out of the posture; turn both feet forward so they are parallel. Exhale; step back to the top of your mat with your feet together. Go directly to the next posture.

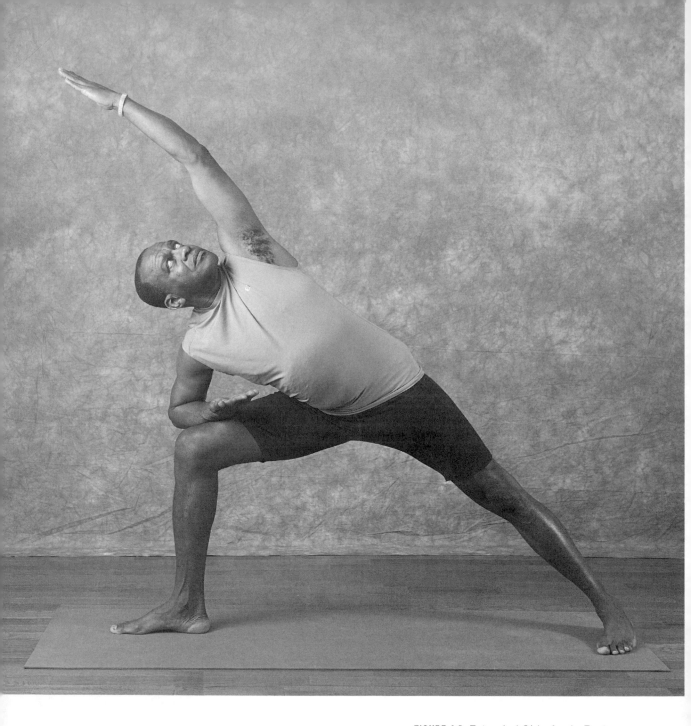

FIGURE 4.2 Extended Side Angle Posture

Posture Two **Extended Side Angle**

1. Inhale and step to the right—this time go wide, making your feet four or five feet apart, or as close to that as possible. Turn the right foot *out* ninety degrees and the left foot *in* a few degrees. Raise your arms parallel to the floor.

2. Exhale; descend into the posture by bending your right knee into position over the right ankle. Try not to bend over at the waist. Rather, sink into the posture by lowering your hips. Rest your right elbow on your right thigh. Reach your left arm out, at an angle, over your head and ear. Put your strength into it. If you can't sink into your hips that far, just do the best you can. With just your eyes, look up at your left hand while keeping your head in alignment with your spine. Do not throw your head back to look up at the hand. Keep your chin tucked into your armpit. Come to stillness. Hold for five breaths.

3. Inhale; move up and out of the position; reverse your feet exactly.

4. Exhale; descend into the posture on the other side. Gaze up at your right hand. Remember to keep your chin tucked. Hold for five breaths. After your fifth exhalation, go directly into the next posture.

Posture Three **Revolved Side Angle**

1. Inhale and reverse your feet again.

2. Exhale; go back to the same right side and the position you did for the previous posture (wide stance, bent knee), but this time, twist your torso to your right while sinking and extending it slightly forward. Place the back of your left arm (the triceps muscle) on the outside of your right thigh, then bring your palms together and push them into one another. Look back in the direction you are twisting. Try to sink into the posture, working to make the right thigh parallel to the floor. Find stillness. Don't fidget. Hold for five breaths.

3. Inhale; move up and out of the posture; reverse your feet precisely.

4. Exhale; descend into the posture on the other side; look back in the direction you are twisting. Hold for five breaths.

5. Inhale, move up and out of the posture, and square yourself off (making your feet parallel again). Exhale; step back to the top of your mat, feet together. Go directly to the next posture.

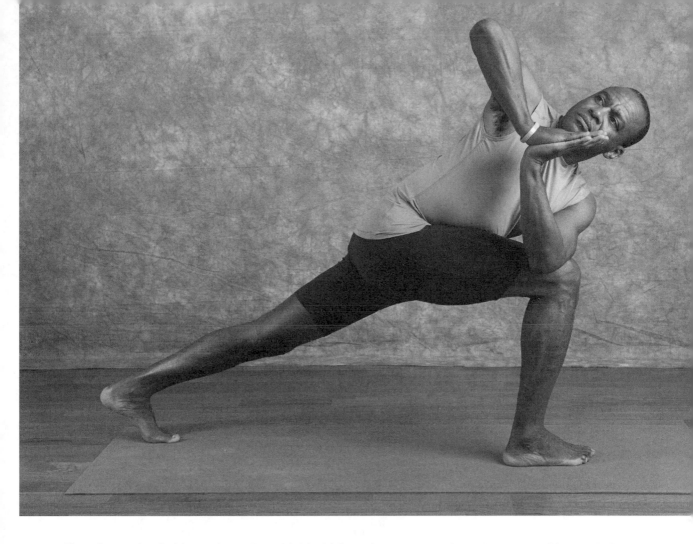

Note: In revolved side angle posture (right side), make an effort to gently twist as far around as you can, trying to move first the back of the left arm, then the left shoulder, as close to the right knee as possible. If you have your palms pressing into one another, this will give you some leverage to work on the twist and open the right shoulder back. But be careful not to push so hard that you shove your knee out of alignment (keep your knee directly above your ankle). You will need to push back with your knee against your arm to find balance. If it is easier, you can lift the heel of the back foot, turning it out and coming up on your toes.

FIGURE 4.3 Revolved Side Angle Posture

Posture Four Expanded Leg Forward Bend A

1. Inhale; step to the right as in the last posture, taking your feet five feet apart. As you step, take your arms out to the sides, parallel to the floor. This time keep your feet parallel. Check and make sure they are. Tighten your thighs and keep them that way.

2. Exhale; bend your elbows slightly and interlace your hands behind your back. Press your wrists together. If you have tight pectoralis (front of shoulders) muscles, this will be difficult. You have probably worked really hard to get your pecs strong—that's good. So don't get mad at them now. Just do the best you can. They can stretch out a little and still be strong.

3. Inhale; straighten your arms as best you can. Put your strength into it. Keep the wrists touching, pressing them together. Stretch back a little, opening your chest and heart center. Drop your tailbone and keep your pelvis level.

4. Exhale; bend forward, tipping the pelvis forward and lifting the tailbone, taking your hands over your head. Keep your thighs contracted! Keep your head in line with your spine. The tendency as you bend forward will be to let the wrists come apart so you can take the arms a little farther overhead. I don't recommend doing this, as it can lead to overstretching the shoulders or hyperextending the elbows. Take five breaths.

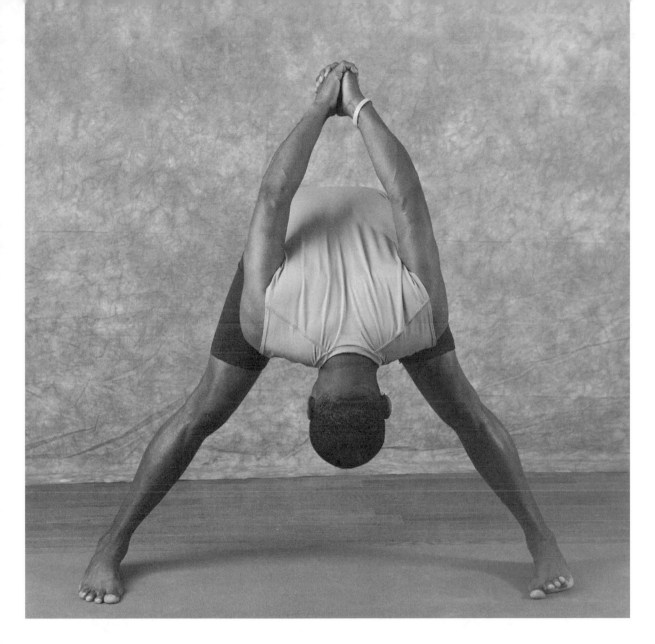

5. Inhale; look up and begin to ascend out of the posture. Exhale; come all the way up to standing. Inhale; stretch back and, keeping your hands together, put your strength into it. Squeeze your shoulder blades down and back, tucking the tailbone again. Exhale, bring your hands to your waist, and go directly into the next posture.

FIGURE 4.4 Expanded Leg Forward Bend A Posture

Posture Five Expanded Leg Forward Bend B

1. Inhale and, with your hands on your waist, squeeze your shoulder blades together, pull in the belly, and tuck the tailbone.

2. Exhale; bend forward and grab your ankles or your big toes with your hands. If you can't reach your ankles because your hamstrings are tight, then bend your knees and place your hands on your knees. Don't bend all the way over.

3. Inhale, extend your back, lift your head, and extend your chest. Look up.

4. Exhale, bend your elbows, pull with your arms—engaging the biceps—and fold into the posture as safely as possible. Let your head relax down. Take five breaths.

5. Inhale; look up, place your hands on your waist. Exhale.

6. Inhale and come back up to standing.

7. Exhale; stand tall, keeping your hands on your waist. Squeeze your shoulder blades down and back, lowering the tailbone again. Exhale; release the posture and return (step back) to mountain posture at the top of your mat.

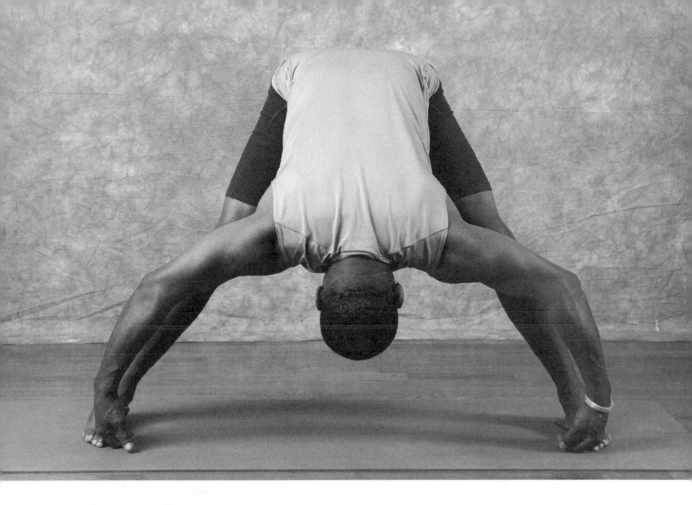

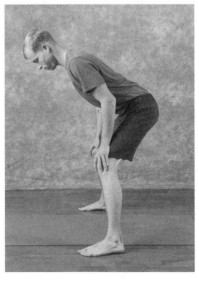

FIGURE 4.5 Expanded Leg Forward Bend B Posture

FIGURE 4.6 Expanded Leg Forward Bend B Posture, Modified

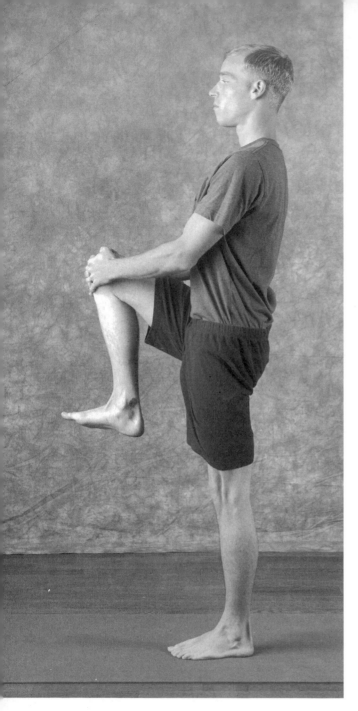

FIGURE 4.7 Standing Knee to Chest Posture, Position A

Posture Six **Standing Knee to Chest, Positions A and B**

Before you begin this posture, find a gazing point straight out in front of you. Lock your eyes on that point and don't let them drift. This is critical for balance, as the better your concentration is, the better your balance will be. Put your strength into this posture. Lift up through the standing leg, through the torso, pull the belly in, and roll the shoulders back.

1. Inhale; start with your feet together and hands on hips. Lift your right leg and bend your knee, raising it as high as you can.

2. Exhale, dorsiflex the foot (lift your toes), and keep your shin perpendicular to the floor and your foot directly under the knee.

3. Inhale, reach your arms toward your knee, and hold your knee with your hands. Do not shift your gaze.

4. Exhale; pull your knee into your chest for position A. Put your strength into it. Your biceps should be engaged. Lift your chest. Stand tall. Your foot should remain directly under your knee, and your shin perpendicular to the floor.

5. Gaze straight out in front of you. See if you can maintain balance and stillness. Take five breaths.

6. Inhale, then exhale and open your leg to the right side for position B. Take five breaths. Exhale.

7. Inhale; move the leg back to the front.

8. Exhale; pull knee to chest again.

9. Inhale; hold for one breath.

10. Exhale; release the posture, returning to mountain posture with your feet together and standing at attention. Repeat on the left side. Then go directly to the next posture.

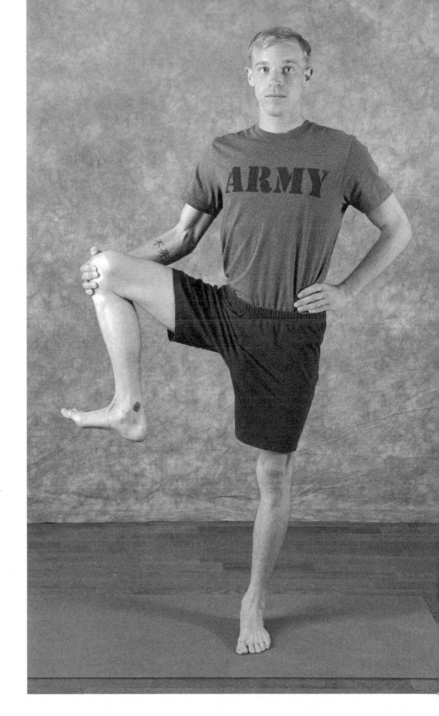

FIGURE 4.8 Standing Knee to Chest Posture, Position B

Posture Seven Standing Half
Lotus Posture, Position A and B

Note: If you are a yoga practitioner already, this knee position might be different from what you are used to. If you keep your knee high and slightly forward as you lift your ankle up toward you at an angle, it will help you to open the gluteus medius, a muscle in the high buttock area that is tight in most runners, cyclists, and athletes who play sports that involve running. Keeping the knee up (and not dropping it) protects the knee by focusing the work on opening the hip before you drop the knee. If your hips are pretty flexible, you can begin to lower the knee while holding this posture.

1. Inhale and, from mountain posture, with your feet together, lift your right leg, bend your right knee, and reach down and grab your right ankle with both hands. Stand up straight and pull the ankle up with you. Tow it up as high as you can, without straining or yanking on your knee.

2. Exhale; pull your ankle in toward your left hip bone. Keep the knee pointed slightly up and forward. *Do not drop the knee.* Engage the biceps, using your arm strength to pull the heel in and up toward the left hip bone (position A).

3. If you are able, take your right arm around behind you and grab hold of the left forearm, using it as an extension cord to slowly move your right hand toward your right foot.

3. Gaze straight out in front of you. Take five breaths. Exhale; release the posture.

4. Repeat on the left side, then return to mountain posture.

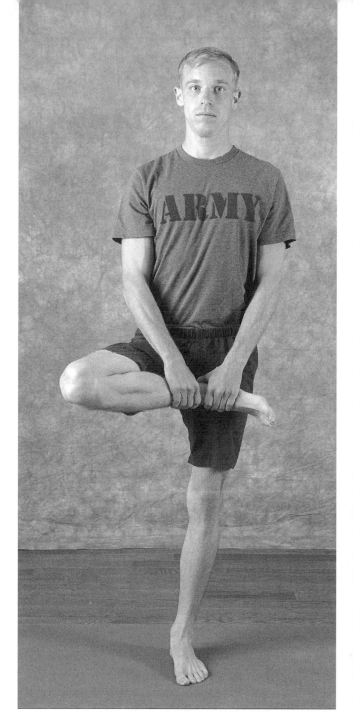

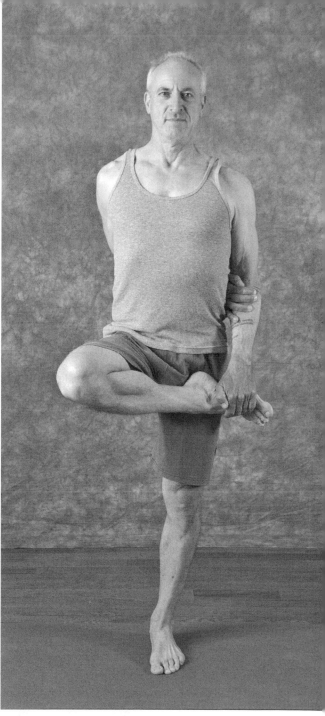

FIGURE 4.9 Standing Half
Lotus Posture, Position A

FIGURE 4.10 Standing Half
Lotus Posture, Position B

Posture Eight **Fierce Posture**

To enter this posture, go through the first six positions of the sun salutation:

1. Inhale; lift your arms up overhead, palms touching (position 1 of the sun salutation).

2. Exhale; fold over, placing your hands on your knees, or the floor (position 2 of the sun salutation).

3. Inhale, lift the head, look up, and extend your back (position 3 of the sun salutation).

4. Exhale; walk or hop your legs back to come into a push-up position (position 4 of the sun salutation).

5. Inhale; curl up into upward facing dog posture (position 5 of the sun salutation).

6. Exhale; press up and back to downward facing dog (position 6 of the sun salutation).

7. Inhale, walk or jump your feet up to your hands, bend your knees, and raise the torso.

8. Exhale; raise your arms over your head—palms pressing together if possible. Lean forward slightly. Sink as deeply as you comfortably can and raise your arms as high as you can. Drop the shoulder blades down your back. Look up at your hands. (If that is uncomfortable for your neck, just look straight ahead.) Take five breaths. End with an exhale.

9. Inhale, place your hands on your knees, or on the floor, and look up (position 3 of the sun salutation).

10. Exhale, place your hands on the floor, and walk or jump back to push-up position (position 4 of the sun salutation).

11. Inhale, point your toes, and curl up into upward facing dog (position 5 of the sun salutation).

12. Exhale, press back to downward facing dog (position 6 of the sun salutation), and go directly into the next posture.

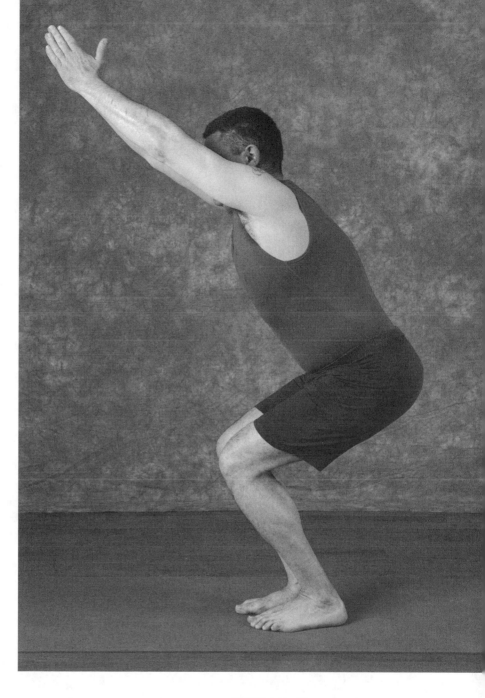

FIGURE 4.11 Fierce Posture

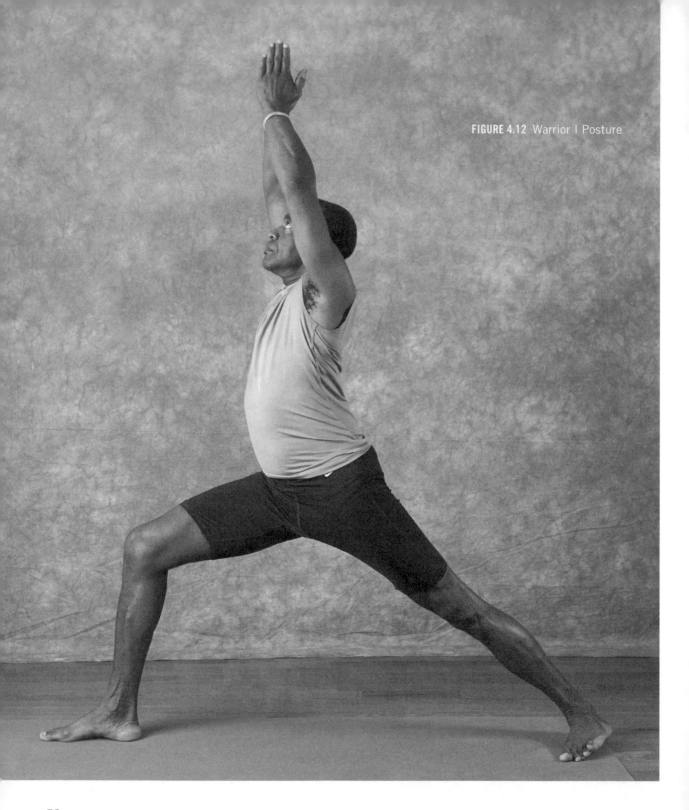

FIGURE 4.12 Warrior I Posture

Posture Nine **Warrior I Posture**

Most of the problems in this posture come as a result of tight hips and tight shoulders, which are common in veterans and athletes. If your hips are tight, then it is going to be tough to step your foot all the way up to your hands from downward facing dog, as you won't have the range of motion. In this case, simply shorten the stance. Just step up as far as you can, making sure that the heel of your front foot is in a line with the heel of your back foot. Tight shoulders will prevent you from taking your arms directly overhead so, as you won't have the range of motion, just do the best you can.

1. Inhale and, from downward facing dog, step your right foot all the way up in between your hands, or as close as you can get, bend your right knee over your right ankle, and pivot your left foot, turning your left heel *in* and placing your foot flat on the floor, with the foot angled in about forty-five degrees (toes pointing slightly to the front). Keep your back foot anchored to the floor as best you can.

2. Exhale; raise your arms overhead, palms touching if possible—if it's not, just make your arms parallel. Remember, this is not a backward bend. Pull in your belly, pull in your ribcage, and tuck your tailbone.

3. Look up at your hands or, if you prefer, straight in front of you. Settle in. Take five breaths.

4. Inhale, straighten your right leg, and reverse your feet, so that you have completely turned around 180 degrees.

5. Exhale, bend your left knee over your left ankle, and repeat the posture on the left side. Go directly into the next posture.

Note: It's really important to pay attention to alignment on all fronts in this posture—the feet, hips, back, knees, shoulders and neck and head. This posture is *not* a backward bend so be mindful not to lean back and compress the lower back. Keep your tailbone dropped, your ribcage tucked, and your belly pulled in, just as in mountain posture.

Posture Ten **Warrior II Posture**

1. Inhale; swing your left arm down and straight
    out in front of you and your right arm down
    and back. This will shift your hips and torso
    slightly. You will be on the left side first.

2. Exhale; gaze out over your left fingertips. Torso and
    spine are perpendicular to the floor. Draw the shoulder
    blades back and down. Be careful not to let your forward
    knee cave in. Keep it centered over the ankle. Drop your
    tailbone and pull your belly in. Keep your pelvis level.
    Gaze at your left fingertips. Take five breaths. Exhale.

3. Inhale; straighten your left leg; reverse your feet.

4. Exhale; bend your right knee over your right ankle and
    repeat the posture to the right as seen in figure 4.13.
    Gaze at your right fingertips. Hold for five breaths.

5. Inhale; place your hands on the floor
    on either side of your right foot.

6. Exhale; walk or jump back into push up position.

7. Inhale; point your toes and curl up
    into upward facing dog.

8. Exhale; press your hips up and back
    into downward facing dog.

9. Inhale; hop your feet up toward your hands,
    bend your knees, and cross your ankles.

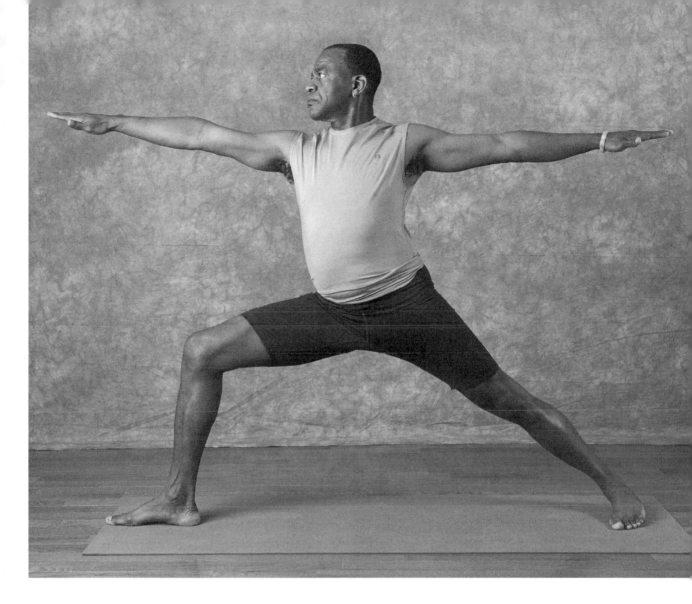

10. Exhale and sit down.

FIGURE 4.13 Warrior II Posture

You may go directly to the first seated posture that I describe next or end your practice here. If you are ending your practice, lie down on your back, bring your knees to your chest, and hold here for a few breaths. Take your knees to one side and then the other, as you did in chapter 3 after the sun salutation, holding for a few breaths on each side. Then take relaxation posture for ten minutes.

DOING THE WORK

Well, that's it for the standing postures. The practice may seem like a lot to you, or it may not seem like much; it depends on how joyful or miserable you are in trying to learn it. In the beginning, you may find that learning the alignment and movements is a bit of a struggle, generally annoying, and plain uncomfortable. That's okay, because those of you who like this the least need it the most! The fitter you are, and most likely the tighter you are, the tougher this will be for you. Since you are probably tight from your years in the service or from years of training, sports, life, kids, or injuries, this is going to feel a little laborious. Hang in there. It isn't important if you like it or not when you start—just do it! Eventually, you'll come to enjoy it, or you won't keep doing it. But discomfort is a part of growth for everyone, at one time or another (as you well know!) and it generally passes with regular practice. As you do more, this gets easier, and the grunting and groaning diminish.

Whether you are just starting out with yoga, or if you have been doing asanas for some time, this may be the beginning of developing your ability to actually notice when you are distracted and what it is that has distracted you. I talked about this earlier in this chapter, and now you can start to experience for yourself what I was trying to describe. If your objective is to keep your mind on your breathing and all of a sudden you are thinking about selling your house and moving to a far-off place, or reexperiencing some unpleasant memory, you've been distracted. And it may take a few moments before you realize it. But once you become conscious of the fact that you aren't *here* any longer, but off in the Rocky Mountains somewhere or back in Afghanistan, it is important that you bring your attention back to the present moment. It is the coming back to the present, over and over, that trains your mind, like a muscle, to be able to do this anytime, anywhere. You pull the mind back and refocus your attention on the breathing. That is how this helps, how yoga works!

Often the mind doesn't want—or is unable—to let go of whatever it is thinking about: maybe it's brutal, it's tantalizing, it's painful, it's challenging, it's stimulating. It feels as if you can't control the bubbling up of memory. All the more important to let it go and come back to the breath. It is possible! Perhaps, you never made an effort to check your thoughts before and keep your attention present. But this is a critically important skill to develop early on in your yoga practice, as it will prepare your body and mind for the more subtle practices that follow in later chapters. I call it *doing the work*.

The standing sequence of postures begins the process of doing the work. These postures start to open up, stretch, and strengthen the joints and muscles. That's why breathing strongly and consciously and getting the heat up is so important. As you breathe and move, you will begin to feel the breath, the *energy* moving through your body, and the opening up and healing of old, tight, shutdown, or injured places. And you will also begin to realize that doing this *feels great!*

Spend enough time with this set of postures so you learn the sequence by heart. Do it three or four times a week for three or four weeks or longer. Don't rush. Take your time. Develop mindfulness. Once you feel comfortable with this sequence and can flow along without constantly referring to the book, you are ready to move on to the next chapter.

CHAPTER 5

FINDING STRENGTH IN LETTING GO

FORWARD AND BACKWARD BENDING

By now you have, hopefully, spent quite a bit of time raising the heat in your body and getting your sweating mechanism turned on. Up to this point, the most fundamental way that you have created this heat (and learned focus) has been through the physical effort of conscious, static muscular exertion. You contracted a muscle, and this took attention, burned fuel, and heated you up. You also included the slightly more subtle method of the ujjayi breathing, which is even more powerful than squeezing muscles. I'm sure by now you have noticed a strong relationship between the breath and your heat level. When you allow the breath to fall off, or forget about it, the heat level falls too, the sweating stops, and you feel like you are cooling down. In this chapter, we begin working with the seated postures, on the floor, and it's easy to relax too much and lose heat. So it is really important to keep the breath going and the appropriate muscular contractions active.

RAISING THE BAR WITH THE BANDHAS

Now we are going to add another mindfulness technique to our practice, even more subtle than the breathing, but just as powerful. This technique is called a *bandha*, or "lock." There are two locks that we will use. The first is called *mula bandha*, or "root lock," and the second is called *uddiyana bandha*, or "to fly upward lock." These locks are intended, eventually, to be "held" throughout the practice of asana and during pranayama practices as well. The primary functions of the two locks are to provide support for our practices, create increased awareness, strengthen and support the core, help maintain correct posture and alignment, and, finally, to move energy *up* in our body from the lower abdominal area to the solar plexus, just above the navel. In yoga, this navel center is referred to as the *fire center* and is the place where we generate heat. So the bandhas help to keep the home fires burning.

The first of these, the root lock, is initially learned by consciously contracting the perineum, which generally refers to a small group of muscles at the floor—or the "root"—of the pelvis, and more specifically to the flat surface area between the anus and the genitals. This lock is engaged by simply squeezing and lifting (or tightening) the perineum. For men, this feels (according to my male yoga buddies) like stopping yourself from peeing when you need to pee. For women, this is similar to doing Kegel exercises, contractions of the vaginal muscles learned prior to childbirth.

Why in the world would you want to do this? Okay, okay. No smartass answers. Root lock is an important way to create a sense of support, not only in your asana practice, but also in the coming pranayama practices. It helps to ground you and connect you to the earth. Really, *mula*, or "root," lock is like the roots of a tree. It gives you a sense of digging deep into our beloved planet and being supported by the earth. This helps you feel centered and anchored, as opposed to spacey and floating around. Having a sense of support gives you the courage to not only move into the yoga postures with a sense of balance and safety, but also to move about in a world that is very different from the one you live in during deployment. It may seem funny for me to be talking about courage to military service people. But courage comes in many different forms, and it is a wonderful feeling to know that the earth has your back when you are venturing into the unknown world of yoga.

The second lock, "to fly upward," is also a slight muscular contraction, this time of the abdominal muscles, and is centered just a few inches below the navel. To engage this lock, basically you pull in your lower belly slightly and lift. Uddiyana bandha supports the breath and drives it up into the thoracic cavity by causing the diaphragm to descend, on inhalation, into a reduced space created by the physical pulling in of the abdominal area. This isometric training for the diaphragm and the intercostal muscles can help to dramatically strengthen these primary respiratory muscles. As a result, learning to use this lock is excellent for anyone with asthma, allergies, respiratory limitation, or shallow breathing that is a result of chronic anxiety.

When we first begin to work with these bandhas, we access them on the physical plane through tangible muscular contractions. However, the bandhas can also be thought of as energetic locks, and can be held in place with only the smallest amount of directed awareness. Even though we learn to engage them through the physical contraction of the perineal and abdominal muscles, eventually we come to realize that they are far more subtle and powerful than just muscular contractions. When they are *energetically locked*, they create what we could call a *closed system* and are intended to move, circulate, and uplift prana ("energy") in both our physical and energetic bodies. Yes! When performed along with the closed-mouth ujjayi breathing, they prevent prana from escaping. Very cool.

Whether you think this is nuts or interesting, it all happens to be part of what you will learn as you go on to more advanced yoga studies. I've put it into this book because learning to work with the bandhas is such a fundamentally important and technically helpful part of the asana and pranayama practices that to leave it out would be an injustice to the practice. These locks are basically what make the yoga postures a little different than just exercise. I will refer to them frequently in the coming chapters.

The bandhas are not easy techniques to get in touch with and can take a long time to master, as you will see. The initial work is learning to hold the physical aspect of the bandhas—the muscular contractions. This really supports the postures and the breathing. Eventually, we want to hold the locks all through the practice. This can take many years of work and requires directed energetic awareness. Physically, mula bandha is probably the more difficult of the two, as it is buried down there in the deep recesses of the pelvis—not quite as tangible as the belly muscles. Uddiyana bandha, the belly lock, is a little easier to get hold of but still requires constant vigilance. Once learned, though, both bandhas are extraordinarily powerful healing techniques, on both the physical and energetic levels.

FORWARD AND BACKWARD BENDING

The postures in this chapter stretch over a wide territory. They are divided into two parts. Most, but not all, of the postures in set 1 focus on seated forward bending; and in set 2, we begin to include some back bending postures, or what I call *back therapy* postures. It is vitally important that our practice harmonize both forward and backward bending. Almost everything we do in life is about bending forward slightly or a lot—driving, eating, watching TV, reading, carrying equipment, hiking, biking, working at the computer or in the garden, and even love making (well, maybe not entirely!). It's also comforting and primal to bend forward and curl up. And, as uncomfortable—both physically and psychologically—as it might be, it is important to bend backward once in a while. That is why the back-bending postures that come in the second part of this chapter are so important to this sequence. They have a balancing and beneficial effect on the body, and help strengthen the spine. They also stretch the front of the body—in yoga we say they "open the heart"—resulting in changes that are difficult to describe and must simply be experienced.

Some of the range of motion required for these postures might be a little challenging. Do the best you can. When you find a part of the body that restricts your range of motion, needs special attention, or is just tight, don't force the postures. Back off and find a modification that you are comfortable with, but that still moves you in the direction you are trying to go. Just as you did for the standing postures, work with the postures in part 1 for a while, until you become familiar with the order of the postures and can start to feel and intuit what comes next. Then slowly begin adding the postures from part 2. The great thing about a set sequence is that once you learn it, you don't have to *think*. That's the idea—to quiet the mind, connect it to the body, and get the attention on what you are doing. Most important, remember to keep breathing. If you can pick up this book and you can breathe, you can do this!

SET 1: FORWARD BENDING POSTURES

Posture One Stick

This posture may seem pretty easy, but it is extremely important to learn to do it correctly with strength and awareness. It is the posture that you will return to in between all the seated postures, to gather yourself and refocus.

1. Sit down on your mat, with your legs extended straight out in front of you. Inhale; place your palms on the floor alongside your torso. Tighten (flex) your thighs and dorsiflex your feet (pull back on your toes using your shin muscles), keeping your heels on the floor. If you are prone to hyperextension at the backs of your knees, be especially vigilant to not let your heels come up off the floor.

2. Exhale; lift the spine. Sit up as straight as you can. Lift through the top of the head. Hold the thighs tight. If you are tight in the hamstrings, you will find yourself leaning back a bit—if this is the case, bend your knees slightly. This is a good place to be mindful of the bandhas and to try and practice holding them. Take five breaths. Go directly to the next posture.

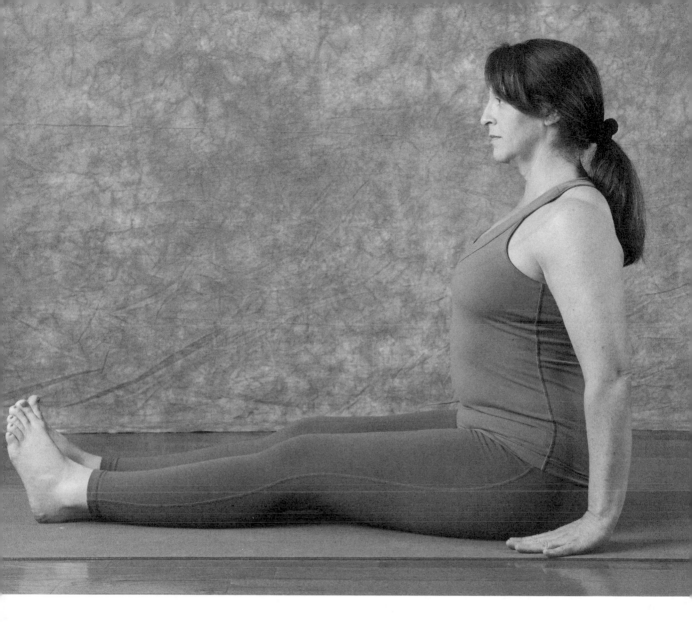

FIGURE 5.1 Stick Posture

Posture Two Lying Down Hamstring Stretch

I'll share a little secret about this posture. I was a lacrosse player in college, a skier for ten years, a runner for twenty years, and a dog musher for ten, and this posture was wicked hard for me. It took me a long time to stretch my hamstrings without injuring myself. If you are really, really fit—for example, a runner—this is going to be not only hard but also uncomfortable. Find the balance between pushing too hard because you are irritated and giving up because you are overwhelmed. Treat the "discomfortableness" not as failure, but as an opportunity for self-care and a chance to pay attention.

In this posture, it is very important to pay attention to the static contraction you are trying to maintain in the quadriceps (the muscles at the front of your thighs). Muscles work in pairs, and in this posture the pairs happen to be the muscles at the front of your thighs and those at the back—the hamstrings. When your quads are contracted, it signals to the hamstrings that it is okay to let go and stretch.

1. Inhale and lie down with both legs straight out along the floor. Lift your right leg as high as you can.

2. Exhale and, with both hands, take hold of the back of your leg, at the calf or behind the knee or thigh.

3. Inhale, straighten both legs, and hold the thigh muscles contracted (you've had practice with this in the standing postures). Keep your head and shoulders on the floor.

4. Exhale, bend your elbows to engage the biceps, and pull your right leg toward your chest. (If this is difficult due to tightness in the backs of your legs, then bend your right knee slightly.) Press out

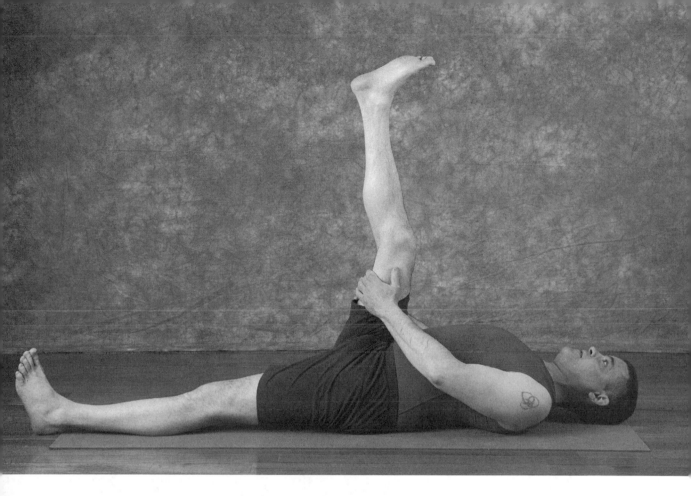

strongly through both heels by dorsiflexing your foot, as that will help engage the quadriceps. Hold your gaze steady on one point. Hold for five breaths.

FIGURE 5.2 Lying Down Hamstring Stretch Posture

5. Inhale, then exhale, release the posture, and take your leg back to the floor.

6. Inhale; lift your left leg. Repeat on this side. After your fifth exhalation, inhale and exhale, then release the posture. Return to stick posture. Go directly to the next posture.

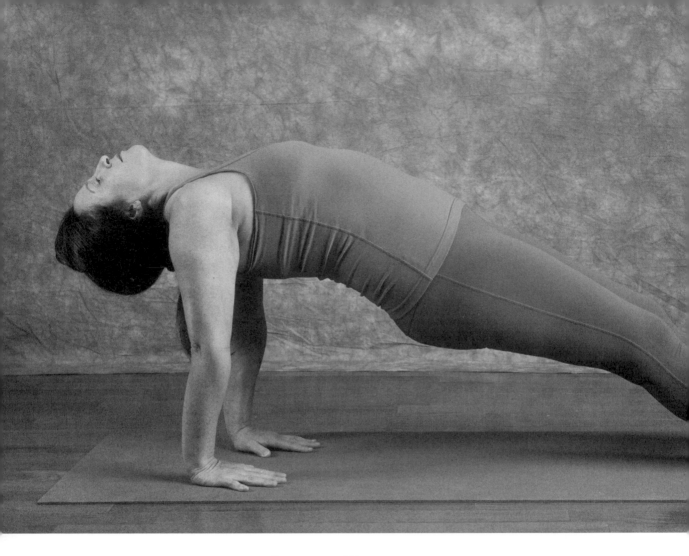

Posture Three Intense East Stretch

If the front of your shoulders are tight, in this posture you
will probably be able to lift up only a few inches off the floor.
That's fine. Do the best you can. Take your hands an inch
or so farther back, then try again and see if it is easier. Turn
your thigh (femur) bones inward, keeping your legs pressed
together. You may point your toes, but it isn't necessary, as
that might cause the plantar fascia tendon (the bottom of
the foot) to cramp. Instead, if your foot arch starts to cramp,
press out through the balls of your feet.

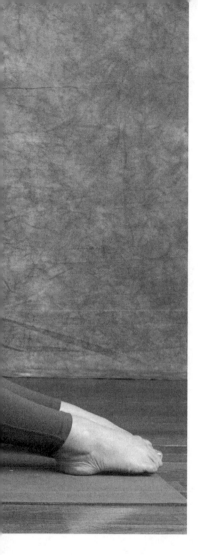

FIGURE 5.3 Intense East
Stretch Posture

1. Start in stick posture.

2. Inhale; place your hands about
   a foot behind you, flat on
   the floor, with your fingers
   pointing toward your body.

3. Exhale, raise your torso,
   and press your hips
   toward the ceiling. Lift
   up as high as you can.
   If it feels okay for your neck, drop your head all
   the way back. Look back. If that bothers your
   neck, keep your head forward with your chin
   tucked toward your chest. Hold for five breaths.

4. Inhale and, on the exhalation, release the
   posture, returning to stick posture. Go
   directly to the next posture.

Inserting Strength and Heat

At any point in the practice, you may wish to pop in some connecting movement between the postures, as we did, for example, in the last chapter before and after fierce posture and the warrior postures. So instead of just going directly into the next posture, you can insert the sequence of movements from the sun salutation. This connecting movement that adds to the flow of the practice is called *vinyasa,* which translates as "to set down carefully." It adds to the strength practice and also helps maintain heat. I always say that when you do one, it feels like you have just thrown a shovelful of coal into the firebox of your locomotive engine.

If you want to try this, do the following sequence.

Vinyasa Flow Sequence

When you finish a seated posture and have returned to stick posture:

1. Inhale, bend your knees, cross your ankles, pull your legs in tight to your stomach, lift your feet off the floor, place your hands on the floor alongside your torso, and then roll forward over your feet.

2. Exhale and step or hop back into plank position. If you can actually curl up tight enough, have enough strength to lift yourself off the floor, and have lifted up high enough, you can swing your legs underneath you without touching the ground and jump back into a push up—great strength work for the core and the arms. If you can do this, land softly—it is a *controlled* and effortless jump.

3. From plank, inhale again, and then exhale and lower to a push up position.

4. Inhale, curl into upward facing dog posture, and then exhale and press to downward facing dog posture.

6. Inhale and walk or hop your feet back to your hands.

7. Exhale; sit down again, returning to stick posture.

The whole purpose of this short sequence taken from the sun salutation is to keep the heat up, develop strength, and reset the body into neutral biomechanical alignment.

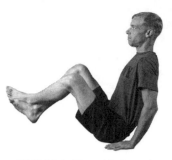

FIGURE 5.4 Floor Vinyasa 1

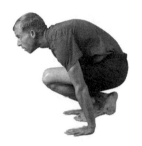

FIGURE 5.5 Floor Vinyasa 2

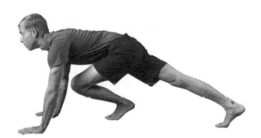

FIGURE 5.6 Floor Vinyasa 3

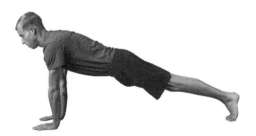

FIGURE 5.7 Floor Vinyasa 4

Posture Four Seated Half Lotus

Note: This posture is difficult. The principles here are the same as in the standing version of this posture. The purpose of this movement is to stretch the gluteus minimus and gluteus medius—the muscles in the buttocks that abduct, or open out, the hips. As I have mentioned previously, these muscles get tight from running or from almost any sport you might do. It is often this tightness in these two gluteal muscles that makes it easy to injure your knee in this posture if you strain.

If getting your foot up into lotus position is difficult, just work slowly and patiently, moving closer day by day. Keep your knee up, especially if it bothers you at all, and see if you can swing your knee around to point forward a bit more instead of allowing it to point out to the side. If your hips will allow this movement, the heel will be pressing into the belly. If not, do the best you can, pulling the foot in slightly toward the belly and using the strength of your arms. Don't force the knee in any way. Do not even think of bending forward. Do not push down on the knee to try to force it into the half lotus position—open the hips first, and the knee will automatically fall into place! See if you can find stillness and breathe, and begin to train your focus now on using the bandhas by lifting through the floor of the pelvis and pulling in the belly. Concentrating on using the locks will help to keep you mindful and prevent injury.

1. Inhale, bend your right knee, and take hold of your right ankle with both hands. Place your foot on your left thigh, *centering your ankle bone over your thigh bone*—a really important alignment.

2. Exhale; pull your heel up and in, toward the lower left abdominal quadrant. Engage your arms by gently, but steadily, pulling your foot in toward your belly. Sit up tall, find a gazing point straight in front of you, and take five breaths. Once you find your posture, see if you can come to stillness while you take the five breaths.

3. Inhale and exhale; release the posture. Repeat the instructions for the left side. Go directly to the

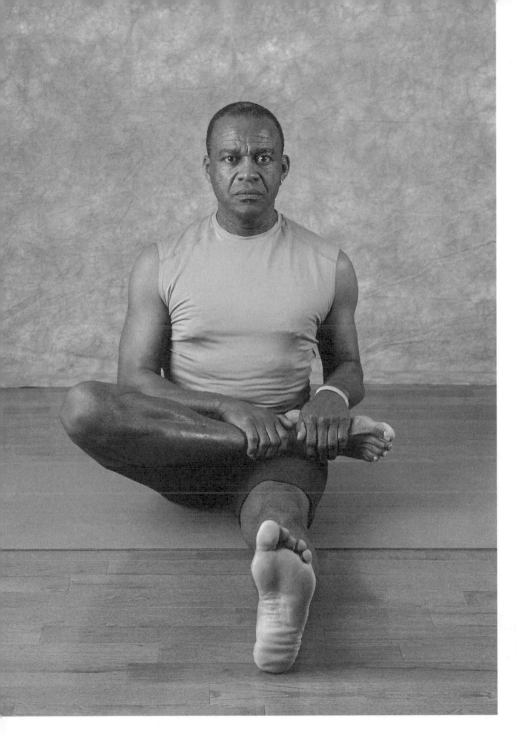

FIGURE 5.8 Seated
Half Lotus Posture

next posture, or put in a vinyasa before returning
to stick posture, and then go to the next posture.

Posture Five **Hero**

Note: This posture can be hard on your knees. You can ease pressure on them and alleviate most discomfort or pain by placing a block or pillow under your butt to lift your hips up and lessen the degree of flexion at your knee. Add more blocks or pillows to sit on until your knees feel okay. If no matter how high you pile the pillows, your knees still bother you, then go ahead and skip this posture.

1. Inhale; kneel down, separating your knees about hip width apart. Spread your feet wide enough to sit between them.

2. Exhale; sit between your feet. Keep your feet parallel to one another with all ten toes on the floor (see figure 5.9)—don't let your feet flange out to the sides. If the tops of your feet are tight, you might not be able to sit all the way down between your feet or point your feet straight back. You might not like this, and it will be uncomfortable for your feet. But this is an important range of motion to regain. If you are uncomfortable or if this bothers your knees due to injury, place a pillow or block or bolster under your butt, which will enable you to correctly align the feet and make you more comfortable (see figure 5.10). Take five breaths in this posture. Try to hold a steady gaze point, straight ahead in front of you, off the tip of your nose. Return to stick posture, and then go directly to the next posture.

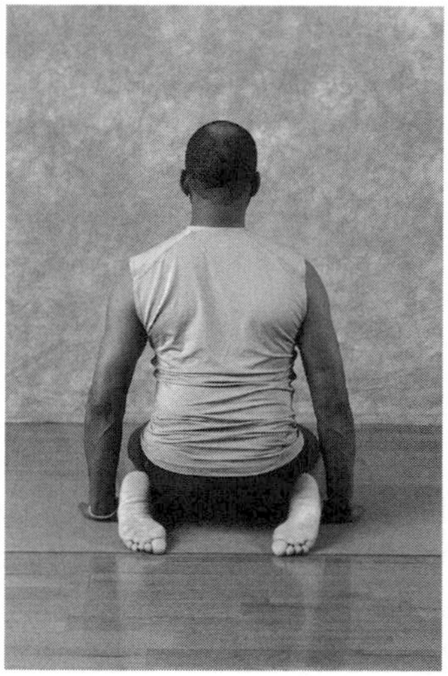

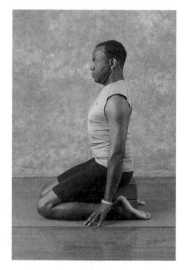

FIGURE 5.9 Hero Posture (rear view)

FIGURE 5.10 Hero Posture (on blocks)

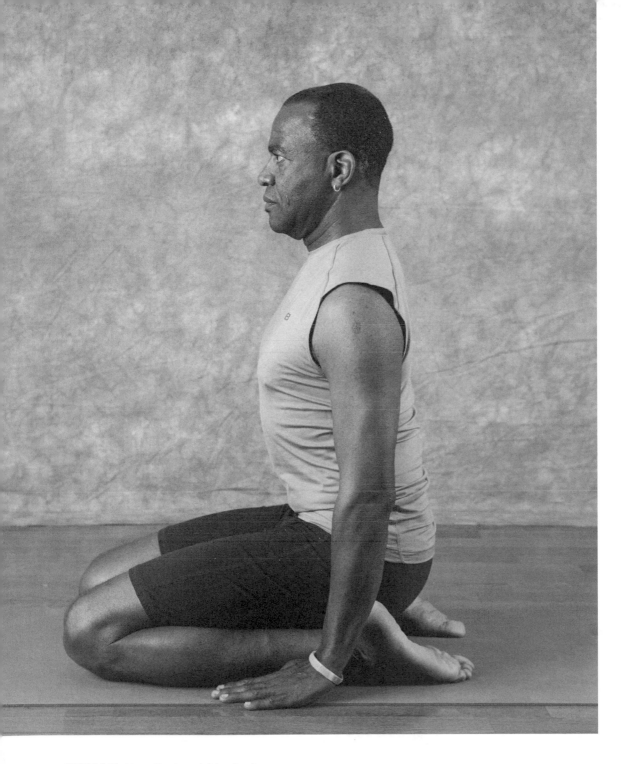

FIGURE 5.11. Hero Posture (side view)

Posture Six Seated Twist

Put your strength into the twist, but without straining, by engaging your biceps and using your arms to help make the rotation. But pay attention. Don't let your ego override your intelligence. Be sure to sit up tall, sitting directly on your buttock bones and keeping your spine perpendicular to the floor. Try not to lean back, although if you are tight in the hamstrings and/or hips, you will find yourself leaning back a bit. If this is the case, slightly bend the knee of your extended leg. This will make it possible for you to sit up straight and enable full extension of your spine.

Note: Read this paragraph before you begin to work on this posture, and then, once you have tried the pose, come back and read it again so that you can better understand these directions. As you start to move into this seated twisting posture, shift your pelvis slightly in the direction you are turning to initiate the twist at the hips, instead of at the lower back. This alignment of the hips will generally alleviate any possible compression of the sacroiliac joint (the joint between the sacrum and the ilium of the pelvis—the SI joint) or lumbar (lower) spine as you attempt to rotate the thoracic (middle) spine and turn into the posture.

1. Inhale; bring your right heel tight up against your right buttock bone, or as close as possible. Make sure your right foot is *parallel* to the left thigh and flat on the floor, and that you have at least a *palm's width* of space between your right foot and left thigh. Keep your right shin *perpendicular* to the floor. I call these three principles of alignment the *3Ps*. They are very important to the effectiveness of this posture. It sounds easy, but most people get sloppy here and have the foot plastered up against the inside of the thigh. Cozy, but incorrect.

2. Exhale; slide your left leg forward an inch or two and shift the pelvis, so that your left hip is slightly more forward than your right hip. Keep your left leg strong and the quadriceps engaged. Dorsiflex your left foot, pulling back on the toes.

3. Inhale, wrap your left arm low around your right shin, and continue to twist to your right.

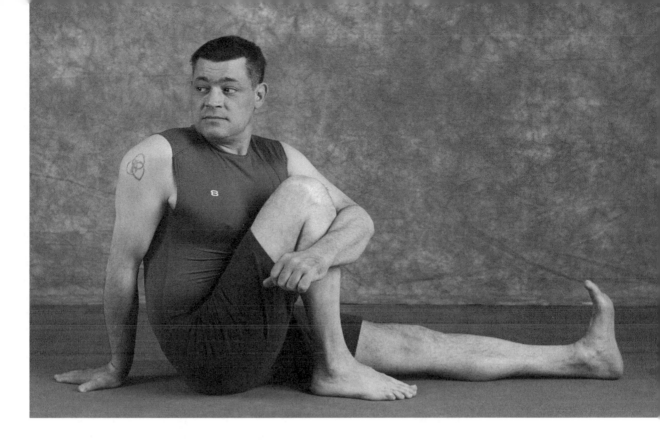

4. Exhale; use the strength in your left arm to *pull into* the twist. At the same time, *push out* with your right leg, so these two forces of *pull* and *push* are working against one another to create an isometric strengthening move. Take your right arm behind you, placing the fingers or palm on the floor. This will help to prop you up and keep your spine perpendicular to the floor and your back in full extension, which is really important when twisting the thoracic (middle) or any portion of the spine. Look back over your right shoulder. Try to hold your gaze steady on one point without fidgeting. Take five breaths.

5. Inhale, then exhale, release the posture, and return to stick posture. Repeat the instructions for the left side. Return to stick posture again, and then go directly to the next posture.

FIGURE 5.12. Seated Twist Posture

Posture Seven Bound Angle

1. Inhale, place the soles of your feet together, and pull your feet into your groin, so your heels are touching (or as close as possible to touching) the perineum. Hold your ankles with both hands and extend your spine, sitting up straight and lifting the chest.

2. Exhale; bend forward as far as you are able with a straight back (you might not be able to go too far or even move forward at all). Do what you can. Put your strength into sitting up *straight!* Do not flex or round your spine. But don't hyperextend your low back either—find the middle road between the two. Don't push on your knees to get them to go to the floor or worry about getting your knees down. They will eventually relax down as your groin muscles let go and your hips open. Keep your elbows tucked in at your sides. You may be really tight in this posture and feel uncomfortable. That's okay. Just breathe! Be mindful not to hunch your shoulders up around your ears. Keep your head neutral—not lifting the chin and not dropping the head (see figure 5.14). Take five breaths.

    Look straight out past the end of your nose. It's really, really important to hold the locks in this posture. The two locks, especially root lock, will keep you paying attention and help to prevent you from overstretching.

3. Inhale, look up, lift your chest, and extend your spine even more, without hyperextending (arching) too much. Then exhale and release the posture. Do a vinyasa or return to stick posture. Then go directly to the next posture.

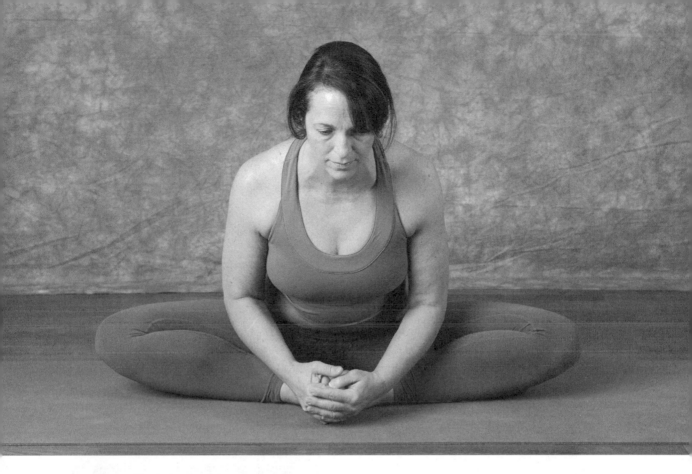

FIGURE 5.13. Bound Angle Posture

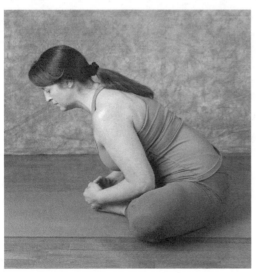

FIGURE 5.14. Bound Angle
Posture (side view)

Posture Eight **Seated Angle**

The hamstrings are very vulnerable to tweaks and tears in this position, if you try to strain or overstretch. Holding the root lock especially and paying close attention to holding the thighs contracted prevents injury. It's important!

1. Inhale; spread your legs about ninety degrees apart or slightly wider. Grab your shins, ankles, or the backs of your knees, lift your chest, and look up. Contract your thigh muscles, and here, as in all the asanas, focus on the root and belly locks.

2. Exhale; fold forward as far as you can. Even as you fold at the hips, keep your spine tall and straight. Don't slump or round the back. Don't drop your head; keep it in alignment with the spine. Bend your elbows and pull with your arms, engaging the biceps. Squeeze the quads. If you are tight in the hamstrings, you probably won't be able to bend forward very far if at all. No worries—just pull, squeeze, and breathe. Look straight out past the end of your nose. Hold for five breaths.

3. Inhale, look up, and lift the chest and heart center. Squeeze your thighs even more strongly, then exhale and release the posture. Do a vinyasa or return to stick posture. Then go directly to the next posture.

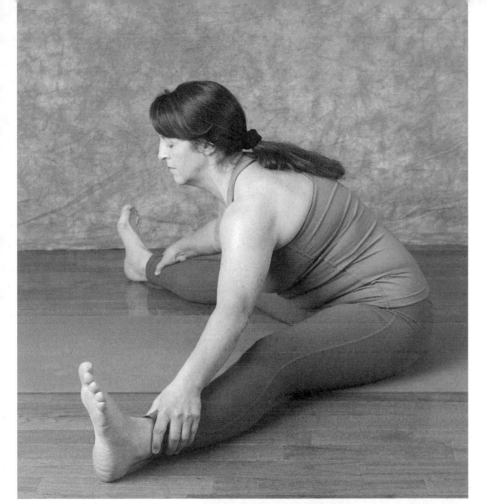

FIGURE 5.15. Seated Angle Posture

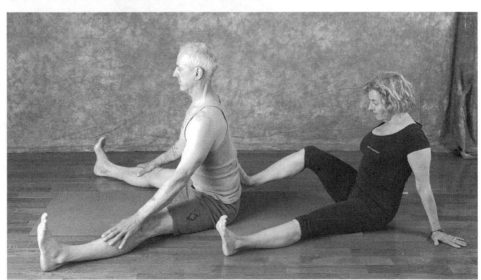

FIGURE 5.16 Seated
Angle Posture, Modified
(with assistance)

Posture Nine **Reclining Angle**

How far you go into this posture depends on how flexible your hamstrings are. If they are tight, this will limit how far you can *safely* take your legs over your head without over bending and stressing the spine. This is important, as this is a posture with a greater risk of injury than others. It doesn't mean you should be afraid of it; it just means you need to pay close attention to what you are doing. As you become more pliable, you can increase this angle slowly. Pay attention. Don't just flop into this.

1. Lie down with your legs and feet together, with your feet flexed and arms at your sides. This initial move for reclining angle posture is a supine version of mountain posture. This lying-down "attention" position is called reclining mountain posture.

2. Inhale, raise your legs in the air, and separate them as far apart as possible, keeping your hips on the floor.

3. Exhale, reach up with your arms, and take hold of the backs of your legs somewhere—behind the calves or knees or ankles. This is the same posture that you just did while sitting with your legs spread apart, only now you are lying down. Gaze down toward your chest. Hold for five breaths. If you would like to—and safely can—go a little farther into the posture; you can take your legs slightly over your head (using a wall or friend to prop your feet on), or perhaps even all the way to the floor. This additional stretch will increase the angle of flexion at the back of your neck and at the lower back. After your fifth exhalation, bend your knees, cross your ankles, and roll up to a seated position.

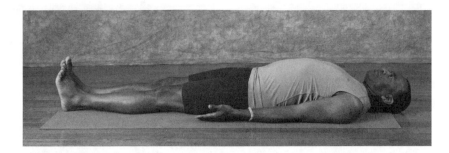

FIGURE 5.17 Reclining Mountain Posture

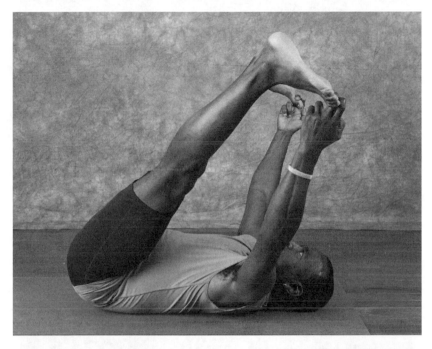

FIGURE 5.18 Reclining Angle Posture

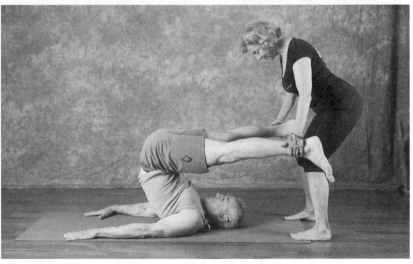

FIGURE 5.19 Reclining Angle Posture, Advanced (with assistance)

Posture Ten
Lying Down Hand to Leg A

1. Inhale, raise your right leg, and take hold of the back of your thigh or knee or the ankle with your right hand. Place your left hand on your left thigh.

2. Exhale; lift your head and shoulders up off the floor, taking your nose toward your knee. Keep your gaze steady and straight. Hold for five breaths.

3. Inhale; lower your head and shoulders to the floor.

4. Exhale; open your leg out to the side. This will take you right into the next posture, which is a continuation of what you just did.

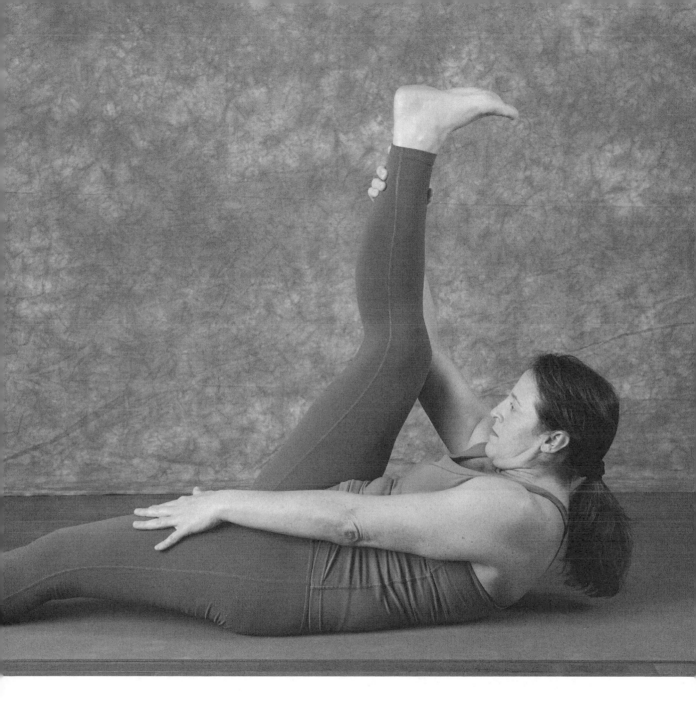

FIGURE 5.20 Lying Down Hand to Leg Posture, Position A

Posture Eleven
Lying Down Hand to Leg B

1. Look to your left (the opposite
   direction from the leg out
   to the side). Be sure to keep
   both legs straight, pressing
   out through the heels of
   both feet. You might need to
   adjust your hand position as
   your leg opens out to the side.
   This is fine—just don't bend
   your knee. Don't worry about
   being tight. Put your strength
   into it and keep the quads
   engaged. Hold for five breaths.

2. Inhale; raise your leg
   back up to center.

3. Exhale; take your nose
   up toward your knee.

4. Inhale; lower your head again.

5. Exhale, release
   your leg, and return
   to reclining mountain posture.

6. Repeat lying down hand to leg A and B for the left side.

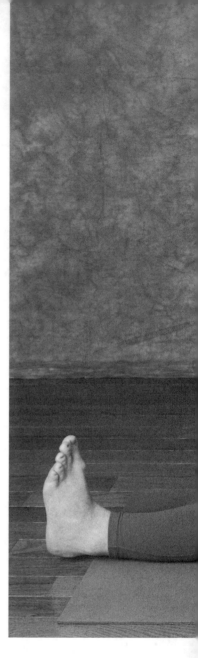

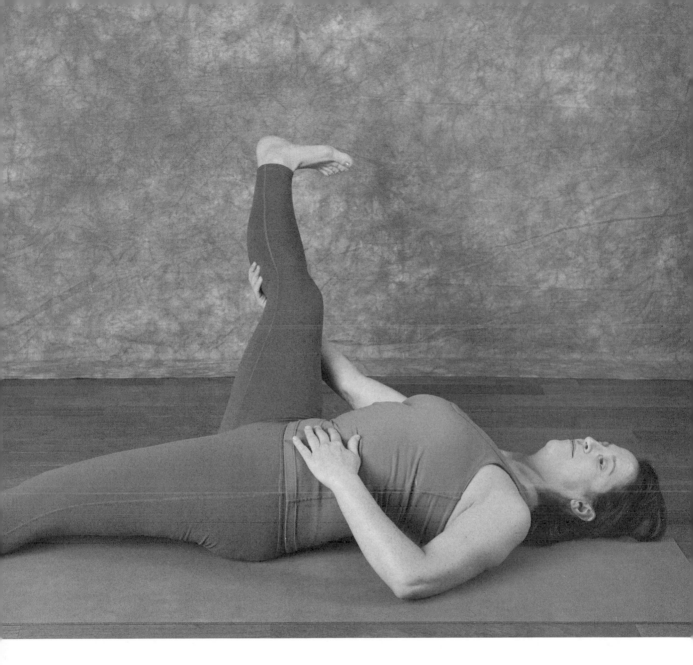

FIGURE 5.21 Lying Down Hand to Leg Posture, Position B

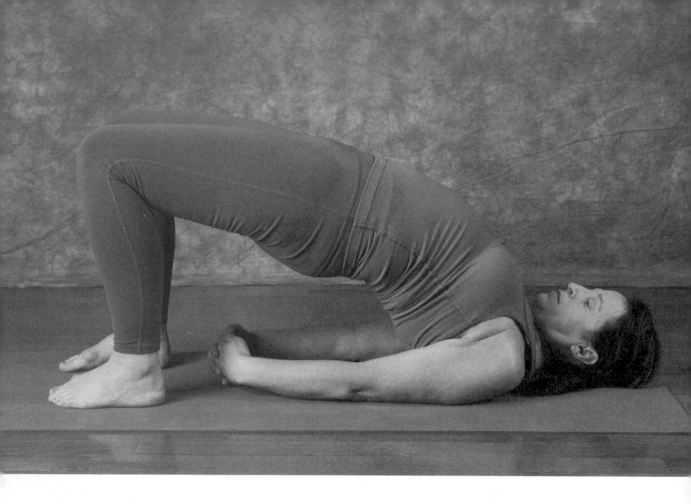

FIGURE 5.22 Bridge Posture

Posture Twelve **Bridge**

1. From reclining mountain posture, bring your feet up toward your buttocks bones. Separate your feet about hip width apart, and keep your feet parallel and flat on the floor.

2. Inhale, lift your buttocks off the floor, pressing up, and lace your fingers together underneath your torso.

3. Exhale, straighten your arms, and squeeze your shoulder blades together, stretching the front of your shoulders and working the shoulder blades toward one another. Take five breaths. Gaze down at your chest, or what is called the "heart center."

4. Inhale, and then exhale, lowering your buttocks as you move out of the posture. Bend your knees, cross your ankles, and roll up to a seated position. Go through a connecting vinyasa.

Once you get to downward dog, you have two options:

Option 1 If you choose this option, your practice is finished for this day. You can end your practice by lying on your back, bringing your knees to your chest, giving yourself a hug, and taking a few breaths before rolling your knees first to one side then the other side, then back to the center. Stretch your legs straight out along the floor and come into relaxation posture. Rest for at least ten minutes.

Your objective is to develop both mental and physical endurance, so every day you will start from the beginning (sun salutations) and build, going as far as you can.

Option 2 If you have been practicing for a while, then you can continue on to set 2; in that case, from your last downward facing dog, inhale and come forward into high plank, then exhale and lower down to the floor, resting on your tummy. This will take you to the next posture.

SET 2: BACKWARD BENDING POSTURES

Remember, you can't just pick up today where you left off yesterday. You need to start your practice from the beginning every day: go back through the sun salutations, the standing postures, and set 1 (the forward bending postures). Set 2 is a continuation of the previous postures. You either stop after set 1 and close out, or you keep going into the following postures.

Posture Thirteen Locust A

1. Start by lying on your belly. Inhale; place your arms along your sides, palms facing up, feet together, chin on the floor.

2. Exhale; raise your head, shoulders, and legs into the air. Keep your legs and feet together. Press the backs of the hands down into the floor. Keep your head neutral. Check your bandhas! As you hold the locks—the floor of the pelvis contracted and the belly pulled in—don't squeeze your buttock muscles; instead think about turning your thigh bones in toward one another. This opens up the sacroiliac joint and relieves compression in the lower back. Hold for five breaths. Fix your eyes steadily on a point straight in front of you. After your fifth exhalation, go directly into locust B posture, unless you need a break between these two—in which case, inhale, then exhale, and release. Reposition your hands, as described for the next posture, and go on.

FIGURE 5.23 Locust A Posture

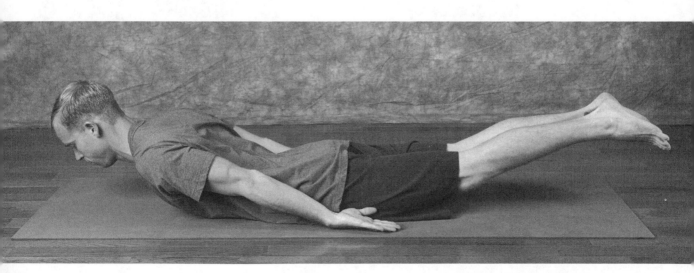

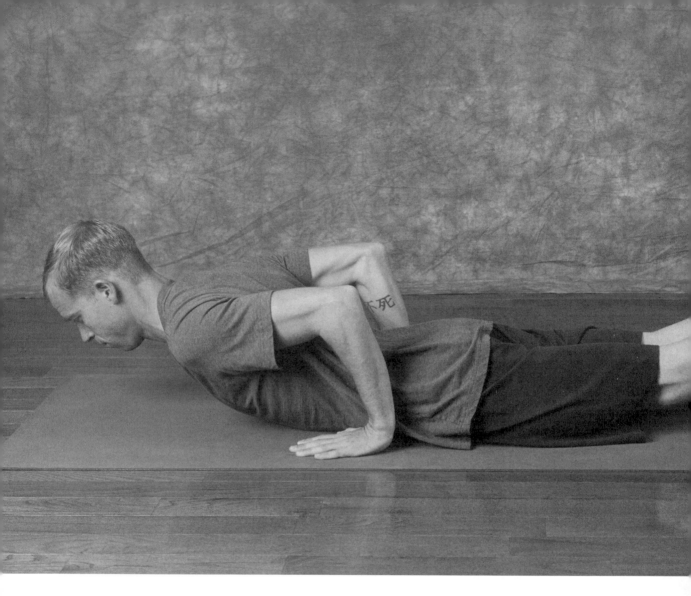

Posture Fourteen: Locust B

1. Inhale, and, if possible without coming down from locust A posture, shift your hand position. Bend your elbows, place your hands flat on the floor with fingers pointing forward, and then slide your hands until your wrists are directly under your elbows, so you look like a grasshopper. Everything else stays the same.

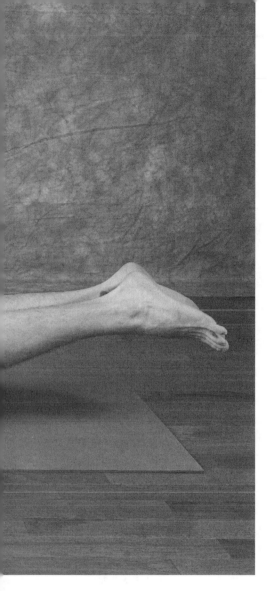

FIGURE 5.24 Locust B Posture

2. Exhale; settle in with the legs and torso still lifted. If you came back down to the floor after locust A, then lift back up again into this posture. Your gazing point is the same as in locust A—straight ahead. Find stillness. Remember to hold the bandhas, with the perineum lifted and the belly pulled in and up toward the spine. It is easy to forget once you begin back bending, but it becomes even more important to hold the belly in as it helps to lengthen the spine and prevents excess compression in the lower back. Take five breaths. Exhale and release the posture.

3. Inhale and go directly into upward facing dog posture.

4. Exhale, press back into downward facing dog posture, and go directly into the next posture.

Posture Fifteen Camel

1. Inhale, kneel down, and come into hero posture (see figures 5.9 through 5.11), separating your knees about hip width apart. Spread your feet wide enough to sit between them.

2. Exhale; sit down between your feet. Remember, if the tops of your feet or your hips are tight, you might not be able to sit all the way down between your feet or point your feet straight back; in that case, place a pillow or block or bolster under your butt, which will enable you to correctly align your feet and ease pressure on your knees. Keep your feet parallel to one another, with all ten toes on the floor—don't allow your feet to flange out to the sides. If this hurts your knees, don't do it. Take five breaths in this posture. Gaze straight ahead.

3. Inhale, lean back, and place your hands on the floor behind you. Place your palms flat on the floor with your fingers pointing toward you.

4. Exhale; lift your hips in the air. Press your hips forward, stretching the quadriceps, and if you can, allow your head to hang back. If this is not comfortable for your neck, keep your head forward. If your head is back, gaze at your nose; if your head is up, gaze straight out in front of you. Pay attention. This is another range of motion that can have an increased risk of injury for anyone with vertebral misalignments (like reverse cervical curve). Hold for five breaths.

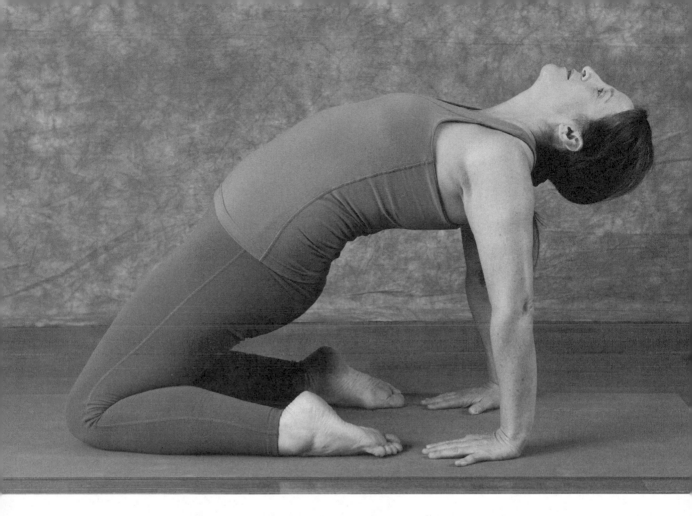

5. Inhale, exhale, and release the posture. At this point, it's probably a good idea to move through a vinyasa to stretch out the legs and take any kinks out of your knees. From downward facing dog posture, go directly to the next posture.

FIGURE 5.25 Camel Posture

Posture Sixteen Horse

This posture and the next one are excellent stretches for opening the shoulders, and can help to rehabilitate almost any shoulder injury. If tight shoulders or an old injury are an issue for you, or if you have had shoulder surgery, developing this range of motion can be very therapeutic. If you have any questions about whether this work might be good for your particular situation, check with your physical therapist or orthopedist. If it's okay for you to do, then I would spend extra time with these. Remember, if your injury or surgery is recent, don't push the stretch. To prevent scar tissue from forming and tightness from setting into the injury site, wait until the healing process gets going, and then, little by little, increase the intensity. Knowing how much to push and how much to back off really requires a lot of awareness to get the balance right, so pay attention. Remember: hard *and* soft!

1. Inhale and step your right foot forward, placing it between your hands.

2. Exhale and gently lower your left knee to the floor. You may flatten the back foot or keep the toes (curled under) on the floor with your heel up.

3. Inhale, place your left elbow in the crook of the right elbow, and wrap your left hand and arm around the right arm, if possible. See if you can touch the base of your left palm with your right fingers. Point all your fingers up and be careful not to hang on the thumb of the left hand. Keep the forearms perpendicular to the floor and gently raise the arms, taking the hands and arms straight up as much as possible. This is great therapy for the shoulders and the four muscles in

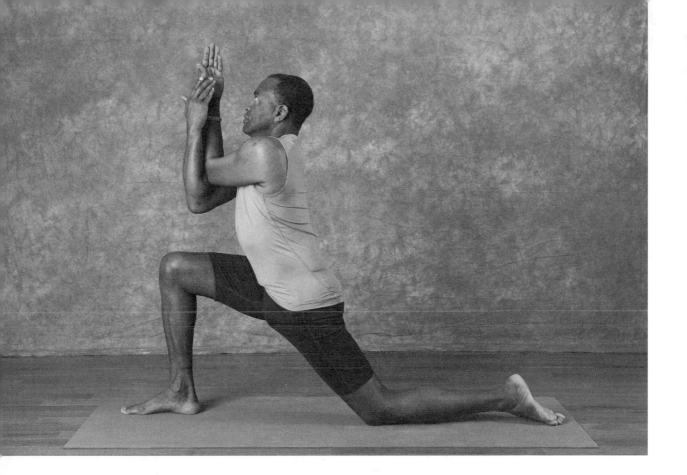

FIGURE 5.26 Horse Posture

the shoulder comprising the rotator cuff, especially the *teres minor*, which helps to laterally rotate the arm. But be careful, pay attention, and move slowly.

4. Exhale and lean into this by lunging slightly forward from the hips. Keep your torso upright. Gaze up at your hands. Hold for five breaths.

5. Inhale, exhale, and then release the posture. Go through a vinyasa and repeat the instructions for the left side, or you can choose to leave out the vinyasa and simply reverse your feet and change sides.

6. Inhale, then exhale, and release the posture. After completing both sides, it's important to run

through the following vinyasa sequence in order
to set your hips and shoulders back to neutral.

7. Inhale; place your hands on the floor.

8. Exhale, step back, and lower down
    into a push up position.

9. Inhale; curl up to upward facing dog posture.

10. Exhale; press back to downward facing dog posture. Step
    your feet up to your hands and sit down. Come into stick
    posture (see figure 5.1). Go directly to the next posture.

Posture Seventeen Cow's Face A

1. Inhale and, from stick posture, bend your knees, and
    cross your right knee over your left knee, folding your
    left foot back alongside your right hip and pulling your
    right foot back alongside your left hip, or as close as
    possible. Be careful not to sit on your left foot with
    the right side of your buttocks. Make sure the left
    foot is clear of your butt. If you are tight in the hips,
    it will very quickly become apparent that this posture
    is rather difficult. It can be wickedly uncomfortable
    and won't feel great at first. But it is fantastic to do
    for tight or misaligned hips or for a tight *piriformis* (a
    muscle deep in the buttocks), so it is worth hanging
    in there. Keep breathing as you get yourself into this.

2. Exhale; fold your hands over your right knee,
    right over left, with thumbs touching.

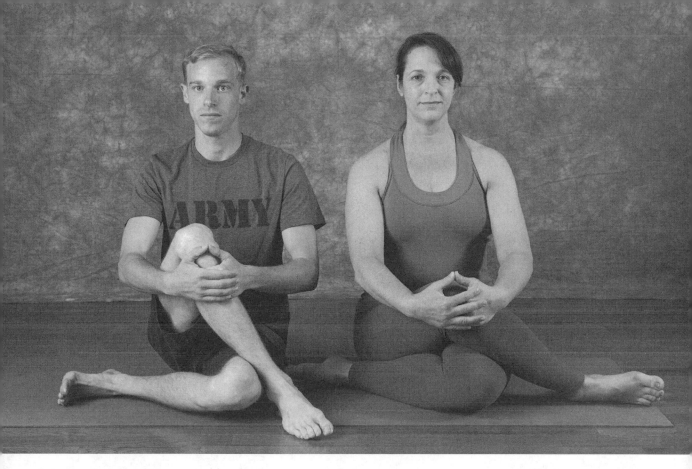

3. Inhale, then exhale and send the energy down through the right buttock bone, anchoring it to the floor. Try not to let it lift up. Gaze down past the end of your nose at the floor. Take five breaths. After your last exhalation, release your hands.

4. Inhale, lift your right arm in the air, bend your elbow, and drop your right hand behind your back, along your spine, with your elbow pointing up into the air. This will take you to the next posture, which is really the same posture we just did, but with a different arm position. You will do the other side after finishing the A, B, and C variations on this side.

FIGURE 5.27 Cow's Face Posture, Position A

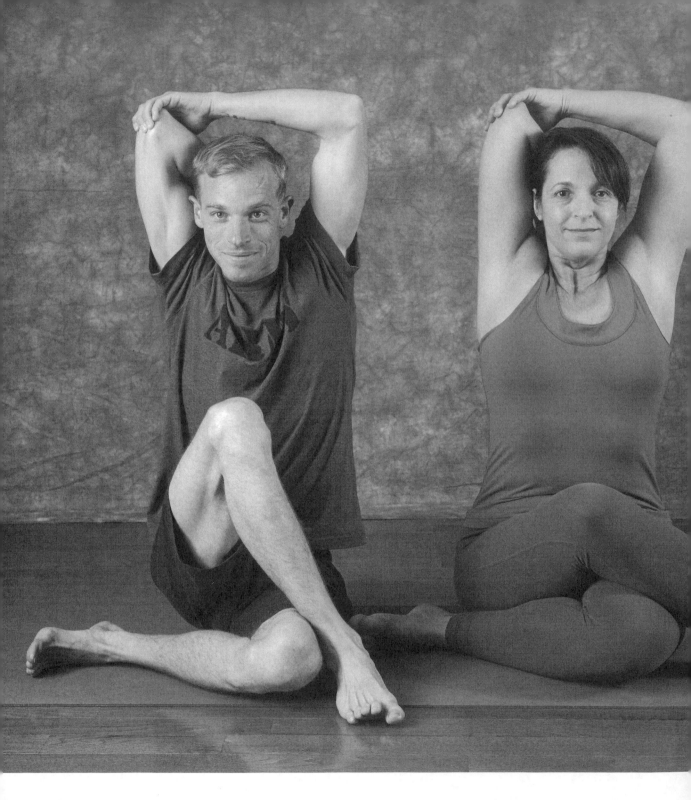

Posture Eighteen
Cow's Face B

1. Inhale, then exhale, and with your left hand, push your right elbow back slightly, stretching out the right triceps. Hold this for a couple of breaths.

2. Inhale, then exhale, and let go of your right elbow. Keeping the right arm in place, lower the left arm, move it behind your back, and go directly to the next posture.

FIGURE 5.28 Cow's Face Posture, Position B

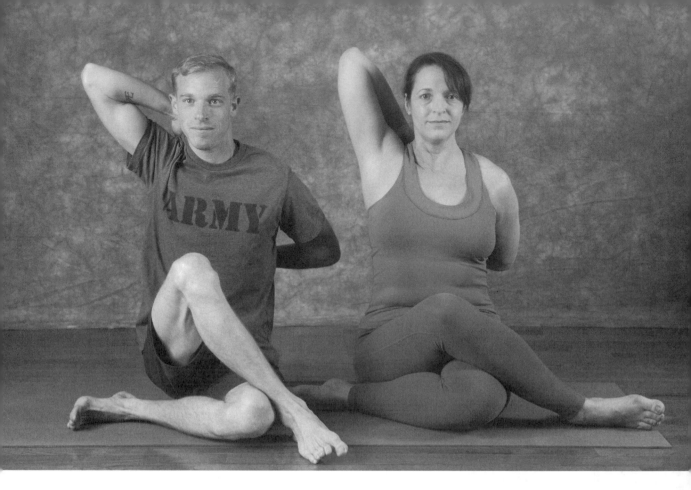

FIGURE 5.29 Cow's Face Posture, Position C

Posture Nineteen Cow's Face C

1. Inhale, then exhale, reach up your back with your left hand, palms facing out (very important), and try to clasp the fingers of your right hand with the fingers of your left hand behind your back. If you can't reach, use a towel or sock or strap to connect your hands, slowly working them closer together. Pull your right elbow back as best you can. Now look up if you can. Breathe! Relax your face! Hold for five breaths.

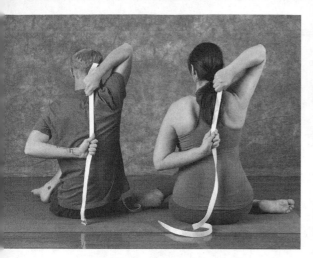

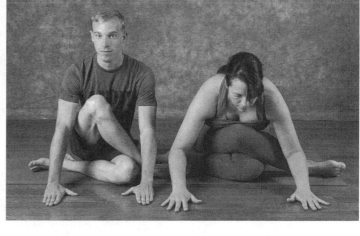

FIGURE 5.30 Cow's Face Posture,
Position C (with strap assist)

FIGURE 5.31 Cow's Face
Posture, Position D

2. Release your arms, place your hands on the
    floor in front of you, then bend forward and
    hold here for five more breaths. Go easy!

3. Inhale, then exhale, and release the posture. Change
    sides and repeat the instructions for cow's face
    posture A, B, C, and D on the other side. From here
    you may choose to simply lie down or run through
    a vinyasa, and from downward facing dog posture,
    step or hop through to sitting, and then lie down
    on your back. Go directly to the next posture.

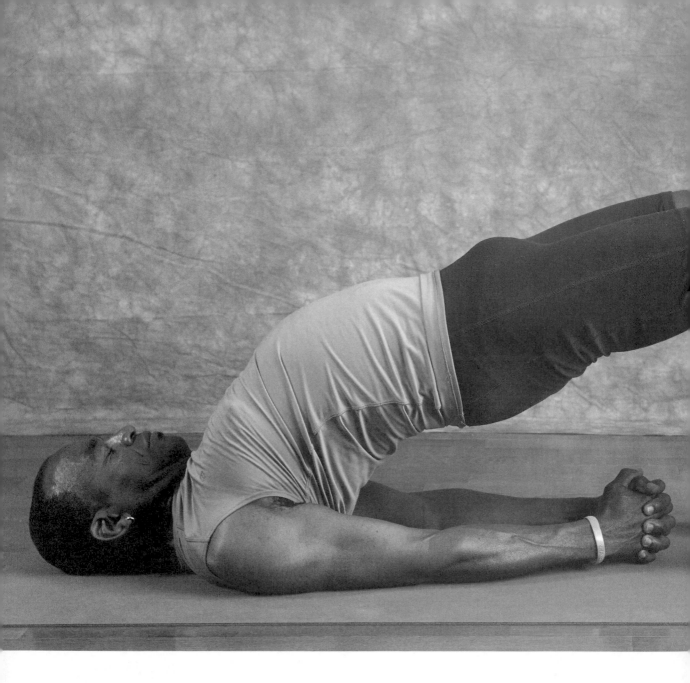

FIGURE 5.32 Bridge Posture

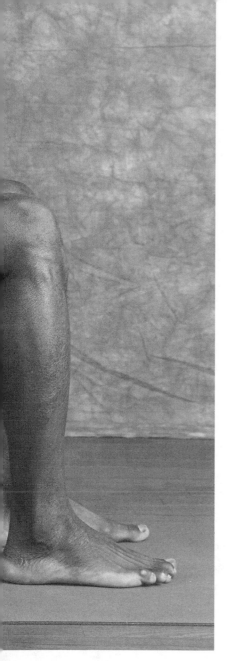

Posture Twenty **Bridge**

We did this posture a short while ago, but will repeat it here now.

1. Inhale and, from your position on your back, bend your knees and bring your feet up toward your buttocks bones. Separate your feet about hip width apart and keep your feet parallel and flat on the floor.

2. Exhale; lift your buttocks off the floor, pressing up and lacing your fingers together underneath your torso.

3. Inhale, then exhale, and straighten your arms and squeeze your shoulder blades together, stretching the front of your shoulders and working the shoulder blades toward one another. Gaze down at your heart center. Take five breaths.

4. Inhale, then exhale, and lower down out of the posture.

Closing Set 2 of the Sitting Postures

That was the last posture in this chapter. From here we go into the inverted postures. If you are closing out here, bring your knees up to your chest and go directly into the supine knees to chest posture. This is, as I am sure you have discovered by now, an excellent, therapeutic position for almost all lower back pain. Here we are using it as a counter posture to all the previous back bending, back therapy postures. Just to review:

1. Inhale; draw your knees to your chest.

2. Exhale, hold your knees with your hands, and pull your knees into your chest. Lift your head and shoulders, if you can, and tuck your nose into the knees. If this strains your neck, then keep your head, shoulders, and back on the floor.

3. Take five breaths. After your last exhalation, return your head and shoulders to the mat while keeping your knees to your chest, and spread your arms straight out from your sides. Roll your knees from one side to the other, keeping your knees high, close to your elbows (see figure 3.19), and your shoulders on the ground. Release the posture, stretching your legs out straight in front of you. If you are ending your practice here, go directly to relaxation posture. If you are not ending your practice now, do a vinyasa and return to stick posture, then go to the first posture in the next chapter.

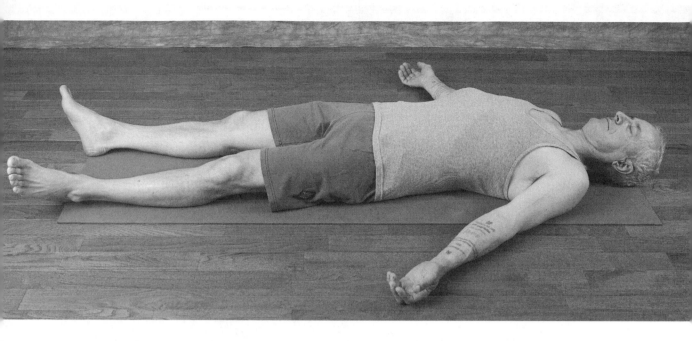

POWERFUL THINGS HAPPEN IN RELAXATION POSTURE

This is the same posture that you do at the end of the standing postures. It is always the way you end practice, no matter how many postures you do or how long you practice. It is very important to lie in relaxation posture for at least ten minutes following every practice. This gives your body and your mind a chance to settle down and assimilate the work. Tension, toxins, and tightness that have been released are able to be offloaded by the organs of elimination, and the metabolic rate has an opportunity to return to its baseline. That baseline may have moved slightly up or down, depending on what was needed; if you are dealing with stress and anxiety, it most likely moved down—a good thing.

FIGURE 5.33 Relaxation Posture

CHAPTER 6

COMING TO BALANCE

COOLING DOWN

Once you get to this point in your practice, you have worked long enough with the preliminary postures and on developing your strength and flexibility to be able to do the closing postures easily and safely. So far, you've been adding postures to your practice just a few at a time. Now, however, you need to add all eight of the following closing postures at once, as they make up an energetic field that seals in all the good effects and closes out the practice. Generally, this group of postures will end your practice. However, there may be times when, due to circumstances, you will simply do the sun salutations, or the sun salutations and the standing postures. This is fine. Do what you can, and in that case, go ahead and skip to the last three postures in this chapter: forward bend easy posture, easy posture, and lifted easy posture—which is not easy!

TURNING UPSIDE DOWN

The first three postures in this chapter are *inverted* postures, which means just what it sounds like—we turn upside down. In addition to balancing left and right, and forward and backward, it is also important to balance standing upright with being upside down. One of my racing Siberian huskies, Nellie, loves to lie on the couch, turn upside down, and prop all four of her legs up the back of the couch. Turning upside down is good for us—we see animals doing it all the time.

Turning upside down is an invigorating and restorative way to drain tension and toxins from the legs, the lower torso, and the major organs, and to assist with venous blood return to the heart. According to yogic thought, turning upside down helps to dislodge pollutants that get stuck in the dark corners of the liver, lungs, intestines, and so on, and clears out mental cobwebs. But before you go to a yoga class and get too excited about jumping into a headstand when you see someone else doing so, keep in mind that there are contraindications for many of the inverted postures, such as handstand, shoulderstand, and headstand.

If you have TBI (traumatic brain injury), untreated high blood pressure, detached retina, any eye condition where increased pressure would be dangerous, neck injuries or misalignments, low back injuries or misalignment, are on the first day of a heavy menstrual cycle, or have any questions at all about whether or not you should be doing any inverted postures (be they in this book or not), *it is best not to do them at all.* Instead, just lie down with your butt up against a wall and your legs up the wall. A nice substitute that is also very safe.

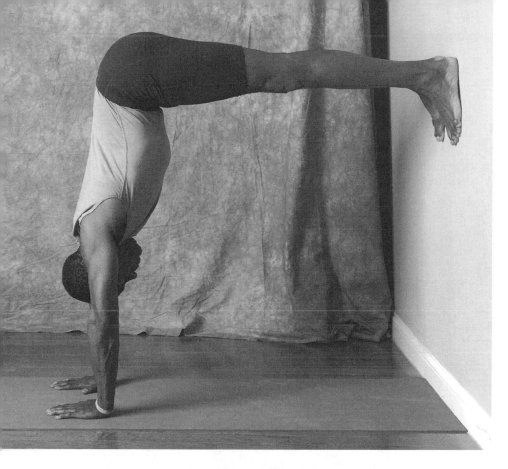

FIGURE 6.1 Right Angle
Handstand Posture

Posture One Right Angle Handstand (Optional)

This variation of the handstand posture is a safe and great upside-down posture that develops strength and offers all the benefits of an inverted posture.

Choose a wall that is clear of mirrors, pictures, nails, and the like, and make sure it is a solid wall—not a door that might inadvertently open, a glass window, or anything flimsy that might tip over and cause you to fall. You need solid support here. If you are tight in the shoulders, this posture will be a little difficult as it will be hard for you to open the shoulders all the way and stack the torso over the arms. As you develop more flexibility in your shoulders—to match the strength that you undoubtedly have—this posture will become easier.

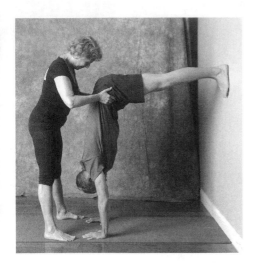

FIGURE 6.2 Supported Right Angle Handstand Posture

1. Drag your mat over to a sturdy wall and place it perpendicular to the wall. Sit with your back to the wall, with your butt right up against it (touching it!), and your legs out straight. Make a note of exactly where the heels of your feet come to on the mat. Then crawl on to your hands and knees (with your butt still toward the wall) and put the heels of your hands where the heels of your feet were.

2. Inhale and come into downward facing dog posture. It will be a little short. That's okay.

3. Exhale and walk your feet up the wall until you come into a right angle. The most common mistakes people make here are: their hands are too far from the wall so their butt isn't over their head, and they take their feet up too high. Pay attention. Get a buddy to check you out or perhaps to stand in front of you and hold your hips (at the hip bone) and support you as you go up. (This posture isn't called "right angle" for nothing. You want your body to form a 90 degree angle at the hips. This means the torso is perpendicular to the floor and the legs are parallel!)

4. Once you feel confident and comfortable, try taking one leg up in the air at a time. Don't take up both legs, even if a friend is helping you. Gaze at a point on the floor between your hands. Take five to ten breaths here.

5. Come down one leg at a time and kneel for a few breaths to recover from being upside down. (Don't pop right up to standing.) Then get up and return your mat to its original place, go through a sun salutation to downward facing dog posture, and then hop through to stick posture. Go to the next posture.

Posture Two **Reclining Mountain**

From stick posture, lie down on your back. Bring your feet together and dorsiflex them, with your arms at your sides. Keep your eyes open. This is just like mountain posture, only you are lying down. It is a working posture—you are not lying in relaxation posture! Gaze straight up. Take five big, full breaths in this position. This is your preparation for the shoulderstand postures and serves to get you centered, grounded, and energized for the posture. After your last exhalation go directly to the next posture.

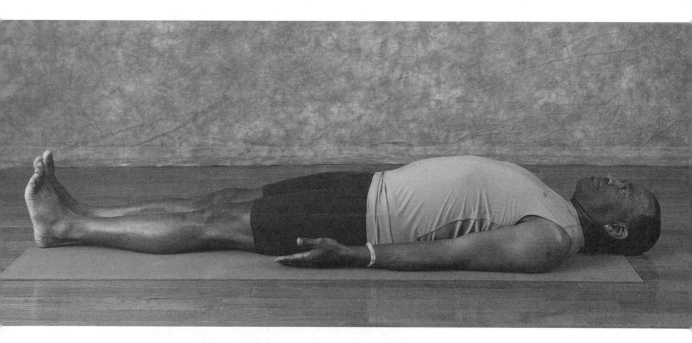

FIGURE 6.3 Reclining Mountain Posture

Posture Three Half Shoulderstand

Note: You will need to experiment a bit to see which posture, half shoulderstand or full shoulderstand, is best for you. If either one causes too much pressure in your head or too much weight on your wrists, or if you have any kind of eye problem that would respond poorly to increased pressure, or if you have high cholesterol or untreated high blood pressure, then lifting the hips might be inappropriate, and you should definitely modify this posture. In this case, place a folded blanket or block under your hips, keeping your back on the floor. Raise just your legs ninety degrees, straight up in the air. If your hamstrings are tight, the blanket under your hips will make it much easier and more comfortable to hold your legs up. Remember to keep your head, shoulders, and back on the floor. Knees to nose posture will follow any of these variations. (See figure 6.8.)

FIGURE 6.4 Half Shoulderstand Posture, Modified (with block)

1. Inhale, lift your legs in the air and, if possible, up and over your head, then bend your knees slightly toward your face and the floor.

2. Exhale, and if you can stay here without using your arms to hold you in this position, stretch your arms out along the mat. If possible, interlace your hands and squeeze your shoulder blades together, attempting to wiggle your shoulders deeper underneath you. Then release your hands and support your back with your hands, fingers pointing up. Keep your chin slightly lifted so you don't flatten the back of your neck. There should be no strain on your neck.

3. Inhale and exhale and straighten your legs. Look straight up in the air. Hold here for ten breaths. After your last exhalation, go directly into the knees to nose posture.

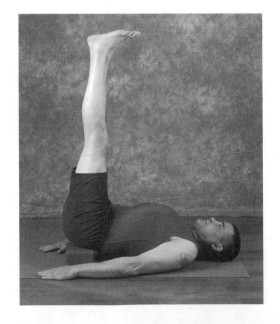

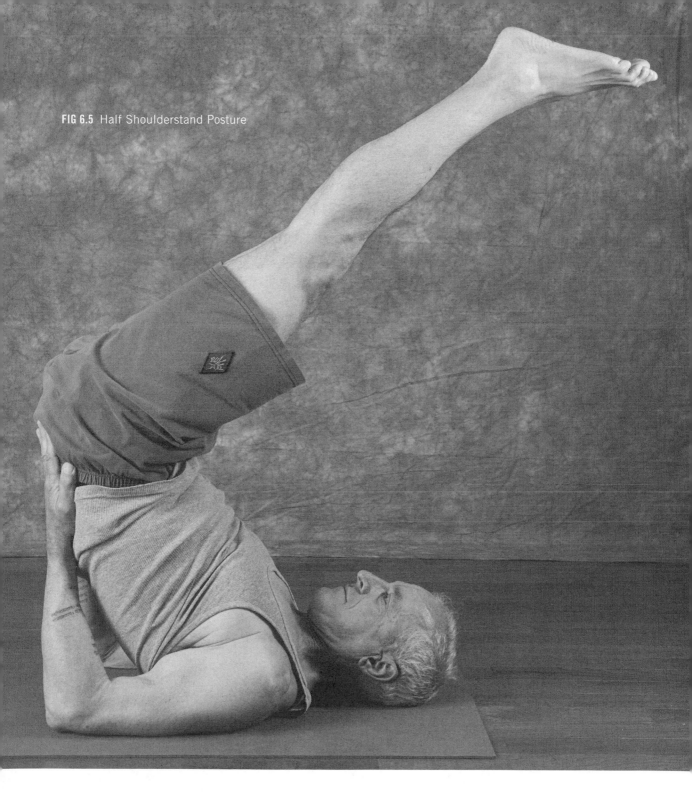

FIG 6.5 Half Shoulderstand Posture

FIGURE 6.6

Shoulderstand Posture

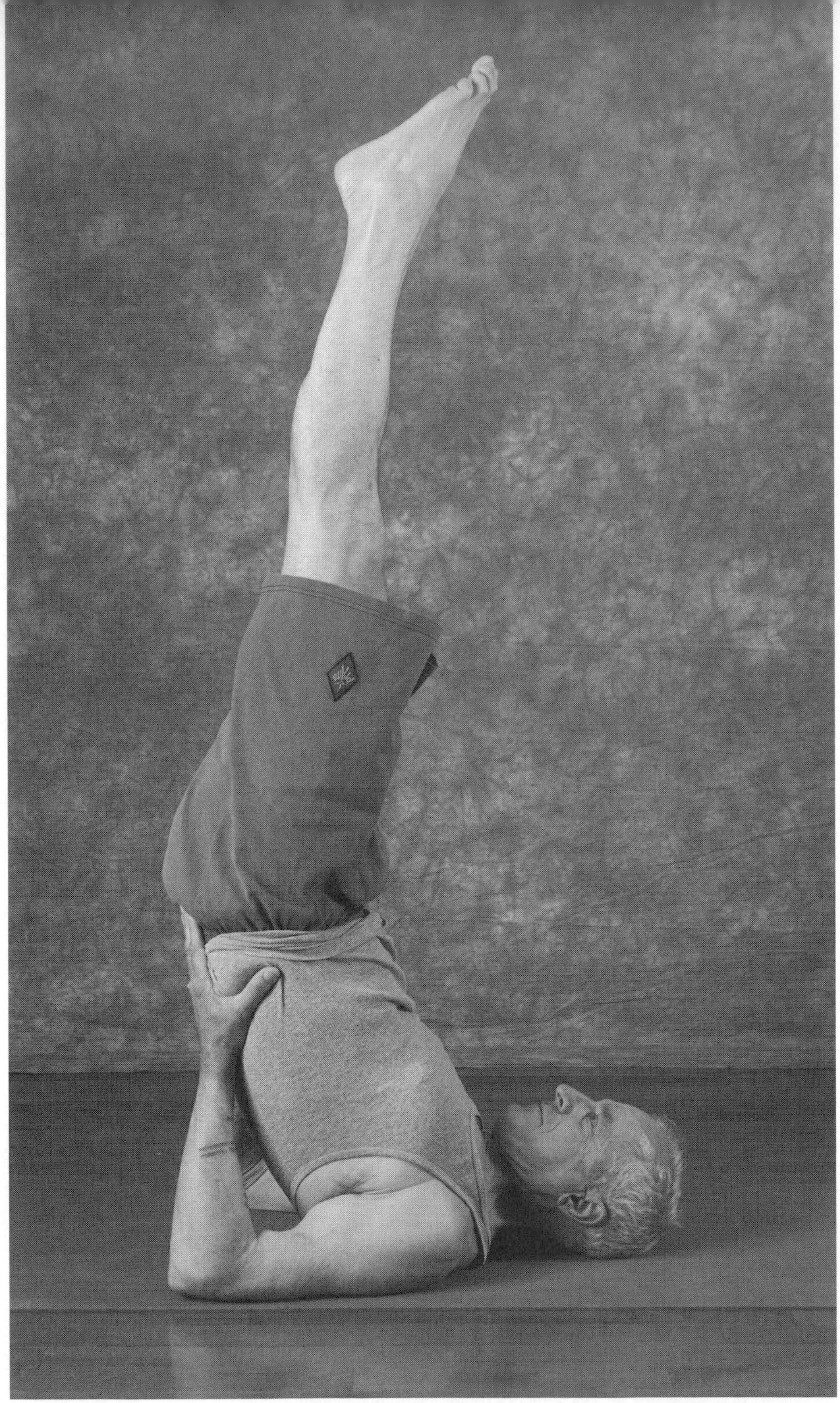

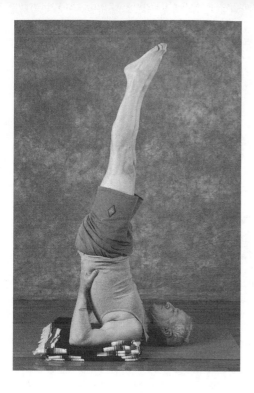

FIGURE 6.7 Shoulderstand Posture, Modified

Posture Four **Shoulderstand**

In this posture, the feet, ankles, hips, and shoulders are all stacked in a pretty straight line on top of each other: hips over shoulders, ankles over hips. You might want to place a smoothly folded wool or cotton blanket, about two to three inches thick, under your shoulders (see figure 6.7). The top of your shoulders should line up *precisely* with the edge of the blanket. The idea is that the seventh cervical vertebra (the bony one that pokes out at the base of your neck) is *just off* the edge of the blanket. This lessens the degree of flexion of the neck and is a safer alignment for many people.

Note: The full shoulderstand is an advanced posture that can be very therapeutic. But, as previously described, it is also contraindicated for many conditions. Consult your health care professional to see if this inversion is appropriate for you to practice. If you are strong, flexible, and healthy, and you have *no* lower back, neck, eye, or head injuries where increased pressure in the head would not be recommended, then you can move into practicing full shoulderstand as best you can.

Posture Five **Knees to Nose**

1. Inhale and, from either half shoulderstand
    or shoulderstand, bend your knees and
    lower your legs toward your chest.

2. Exhale; bend your knees toward your nose or forehead.
    If you are flexible enough, separate your legs and lower
    your knees a little farther toward your ears. Either
    continue to support your back with your hands or
    lower your arms to the mat. This is a great stretch
    for the lower and middle back. Gaze down toward
    your heart center. Take five breaths in this position.

3. Inhale, exhale, and roll on your back, down and out
    of this posture, and come right into the next posture.

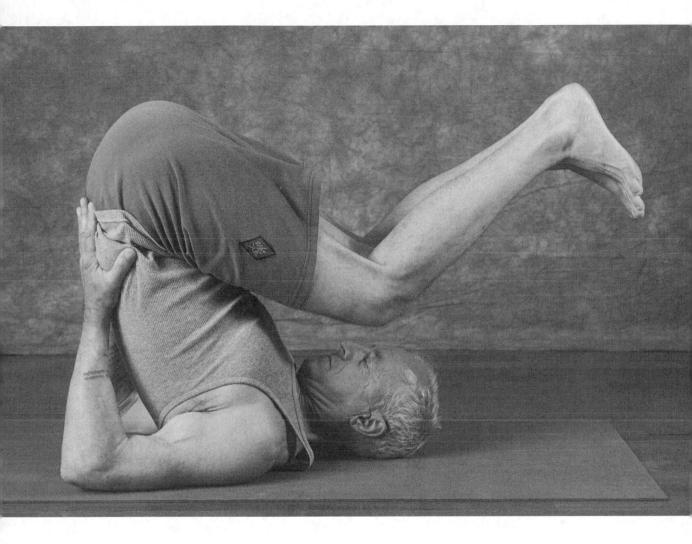

FIGURE 6.8 Knees to Nose Posture

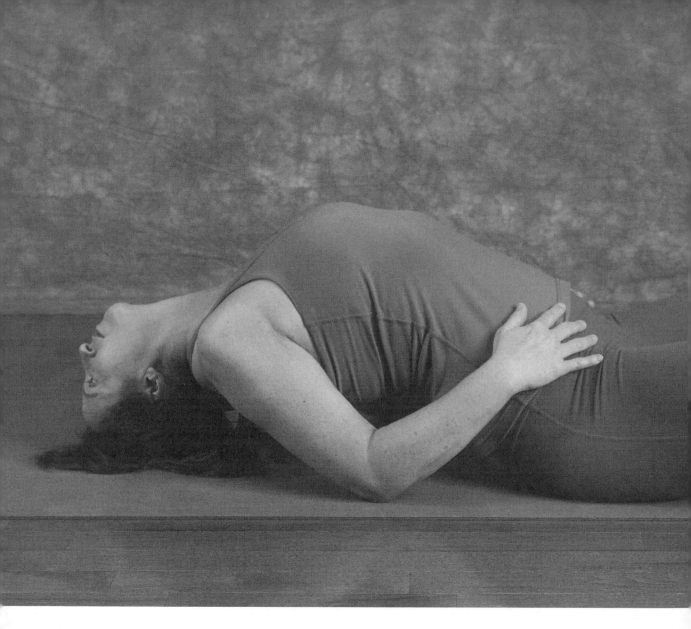

Posture Six Fish

1. Inhale, bend your knees to your chest, and cross your ankles. Pull your feet in toward your groin.

2. Exhale, allow your knees to fall open to the sides, and place your elbows on the floor, alongside your torso.

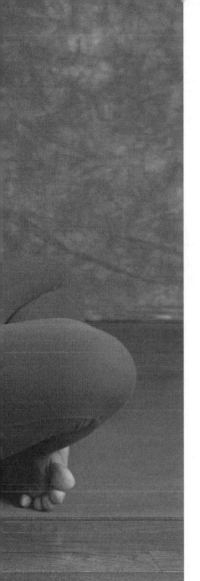

FIGURE 6.9 Fish Posture

3. Inhale and, using your arms for leverage, arch your chest, press your elbows into the floor, and lift your chest off the floor. Arch your head back as much as is comfortable, coming to rest on the back or the top of the head.

4. Exhale; place your fingertips on the tops of your inner thighs. Keep your elbows on the floor to help support the weight of your torso. Gaze off the tip of your nose. Take five breaths.

5. Inhale, exhale, and release the posture by gently sliding your head out, bringing your chin to your chest. Don't snap your head out of the posture or lift it. Just slide it out, keeping the weight of the head on the floor as you bring your chin back toward your chest.

Note: This should *not be practiced* by anyone with head or neck injuries. The degree that it is possible or safe to take the head back in this posture varies hugely from one person to the next. You've got to use your head—both literally and figuratively. Using the neck muscles to help lift the chest will build strength, provided you don't have neck misalignment or injury. You need to pay attention to your range of motion and what is possible.

6. At this point you need to decide if you are going to do the next posture or skip it. If you decide you want to do it, go directly into it from fish posture, without sliding your head out of position. Otherwise, finish the posture as indicated in step 5, and then go directly to low plank posture.

Posture Seven Extended Leg (Optional)

1. Inhale, uncross your feet, and bring your knees and feet together, keeping your head in the same position.

2. Exhale, lift your feet off the floor, move your knees toward your chest, and then extend your legs straight into the air at about a 45 degree angle. Stretch out your arms in front of you and bring your palms together over your legs. It is very important to tuck the tailbone and take the arch out of your lower back. If you drop your tailbone, pull the belly in, and concentrate on using the abdominal muscles to hold the legs off the floor, you can stay here forever. Look off the tip of your nose. Take five breaths.

3. After your last exhalation, release the posture by bending your knees, putting your feet down, and sliding your head gently out of the posture, moving your chin toward your chest. If you like, you can also use your hands to help slightly lift your head out of the posture and place it down flat on the floor. Then cross your ankles and roll up to a comfortable seated position. Go through a vinyasa or just come onto your hands and knees for the next posture.

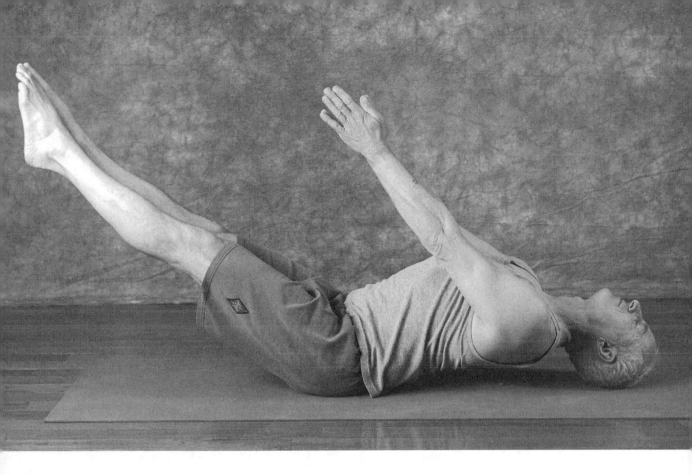

FIGURE 6.10 Extended Leg Posture

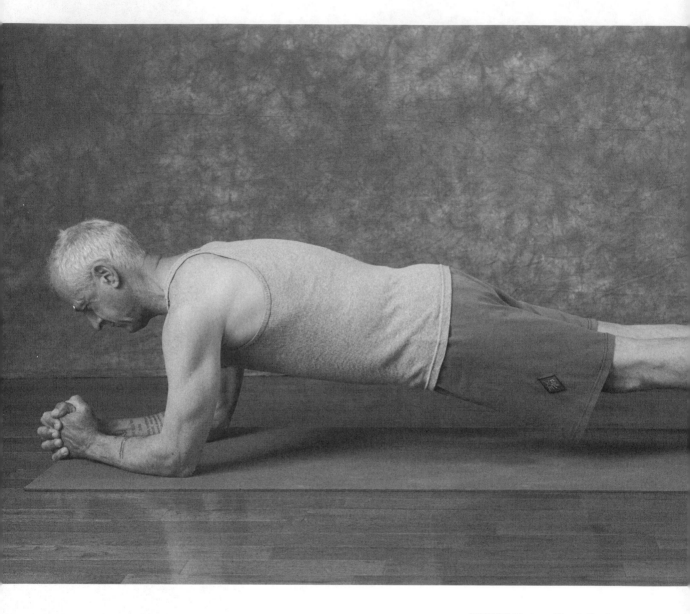

FIGURE 6.11 Low Plank Posture

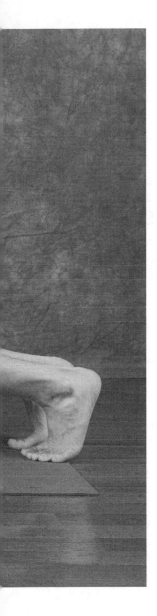

Posture Eight **Low Plank**

1. Inhale; place your forearms
    on the floor, with your elbows
    about shoulder width apart,
    and interlace your hands.

2. Exhale, walk your feet straight
    back, press out through your heels,
    and come into low plank posture.
    Engage your quadriceps and lift the
    belly up toward the spine. Don't
    sag. Hold for ten breaths. This is a
    great strengthening posture for belly
    and shoulder muscles. I encourage
    my students to feel welcome to
    practice this anytime, every day!

THE THREE CLOSING LOTUS POSTURES

The following three postures—forward bend easy posture, easy posture, and lifted easy posture—comprise the end of your practice. They are thought to seal in all the good effects of your work. They should run together seamlessly until the last breath of the third posture. When you have limited time, you can simply do sun salutations and these three postures. This is thought to be minimum daily practice. These three postures (which are modifications of a classical yoga posture that requires great hip flexibility) are specially designed for athletes who are tight from their training.

Posture Nine Forward Bend Easy

This posture is a counterposture to the fish and extended leg postures and reverses the backward bend of the spine that you did in those previous two postures.

1. Inhale; come to a comfortable, cross-legged, seated position. Sit up tall, lifting the torso, yet tucking the rib cage. Cross your arms behind you.

2. Exhale; bend forward as far as possible. It may only be possible for you to bend slightly forward, or it may be possible for you to take your head all the way to the floor. If you need your hands on the floor in front of you to make the forward bend a bit more comfortable, that is fine. Don't allow your buttocks bones to come off the floor since that will tip you forward too much. Keep your butt grounded (always good advice!). Look down off the tip of your nose. Take five breaths. After your last exhalation, sit back up and go directly into the next posture.

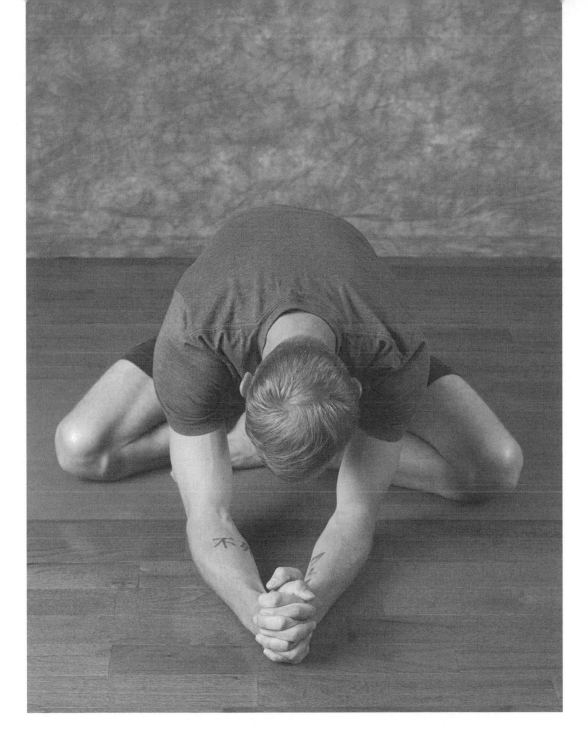

FIGURE 6.12 Forward Bend Easy Posture

Posture Ten Easy or Lotus Posture

This is the posture that you will be using in the coming chapters (unless you choose to sit in a chair) for your breathing and meditation practices, so become familiar and comfortable with it. If you are familiar with the full lotus posture and are flexible enough to be able to do it easily, then feel welcome to come into that posture instead of easy posture. Begin in a comfortable cross-legged position. In order to sit comfortably, it is important that your hips are slightly higher than your knees. To do this, you may need to sit on a firm pillow or meditation cushion.

1. Inhale; extend your arms out in front of you.

2. Exhale; lower your arms, palms face up, onto your knees. Rest the backs of your hands, or wrists, or arms (which part touches your knees will depend on how long your arms are) on your knees with your hands open and relaxed, and your thumb and the forefinger just touching. Or you may just rest your hands on your knees, palms facing down, or rest your hands in your lap, with one hand on top of the other, palms facing up.

3. Inhale; lift your lower back and chest. Keep your spine long and extended, without overarching. Tuck the ribcage.

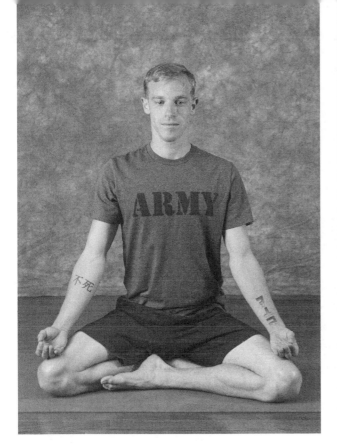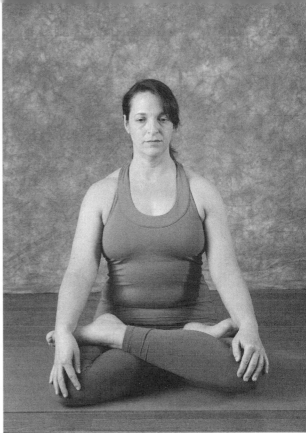

FIGURE 6.13 Easy Posture

FIGURE 6.14 Full Lotus Posture

4. Exhale; drop your head forward a bit, moving
    your chin slightly toward your chest. Take ten
    long and slow breaths, using very controlled ujjayi
    pranayama breathing. Make sure to check your
    locks and give a good amount of attention to
    keeping them engaged. They are very important,
    as we go forward, for successful and correct
    pranayama. Go directly to the last posture.

Posture Eleven
Lifted Easy or Lifted Lotus Posture

1. Inhale; place your hands flat on the floor at your sides. Lean slightly forward.

2. Exhale; lift yourself off the ground, pressing down into the hands and lifting your butt and one or both legs off the ground. This is quite difficult and requires pretty strong abdominal muscles to lift both legs. So to begin, just push down, lean forward, and lift one leg for five breaths, keeping the other foot on the ground, and then switch. If you were able to do full lotus in the last posture, then just stay in that position and lift yourself up! This is actually easier to do than the "easy" version. Take ten breaths total, or as many as possible, slowly increasing the number of breaths you are able to take. Look straight out in front of you.

3. Inhale, and exhale, and release the posture by returning your weight to the floor. Move through a vinyasa. This is the last vinyasa, so go slowly and mindfully, being careful to include every cell in your body in the process. Nothing at this point should dangle outside your awareness. From downward facing dog posture, go directly to relaxation posture.

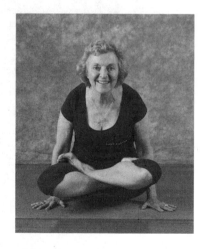

FIGURE 6.15 Lifted Lotus Posture

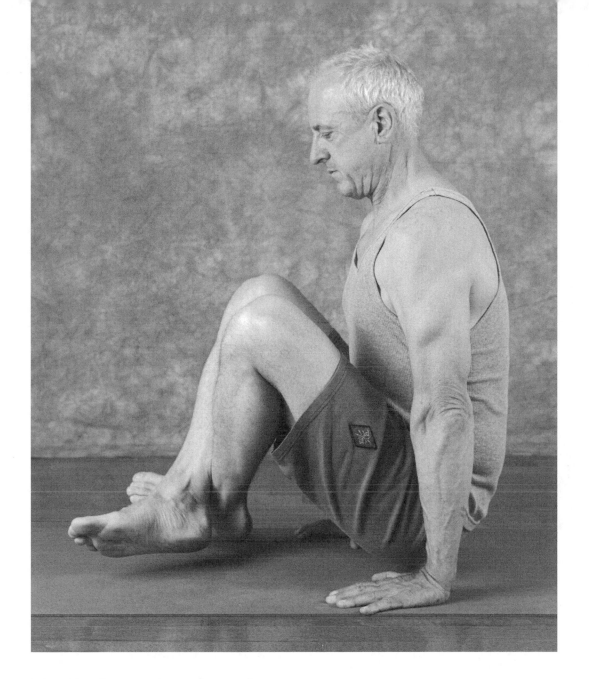

FIGURE 6.16 Lifted Easy Posture (not easy!)

REST: AT EASE

Congratulations. You have made it all the way through the entire asana practice. By this time you have had a good deal of practice with the relaxation posture. This is the final, final posture.

If you come into rest position and you find that your lower back is a bit uncomfortable, just bring your knees to your chest and give them a hug. Hold this position for a few breaths, and then roll the knees from side to side. This should alleviate any uneasiness in the lower back.

Once your legs are straight again, check to make sure that your feet are hip width apart (or slightly wider), and that they are falling open to the sides and completely relaxed. Rest your arms at your sides, palms facing up. Make sure your head is centered and your chin is level with your forehead. This is an asana, like all the others, and should be done with awareness and attention to correct alignment. It is very important here that you don't get chilled, so it is a good idea to have a light blanket or throw to cover yourself, or a long-sleeve jacket or shirt handy to put on.

Take rest. Lie still in rest for at least ten minutes. Continue to use the ujjayi breathing method for the first few minutes, but let it gradually fall away. Slowly allow your breath to return to normal, natural breathing, keeping your attention focused on the breath. Deeply let go and relax. Let the mind share the stillness and relaxation enjoyed by the body. You might fall asleep. That's okay.

This completes the asana portion of your yoga practice. If you are just learning yoga, I cannot stress enough how important it is to go easy and take your time. Even with modifications and options, and as simple, safe, balanced, comfortable, and therapeutic as I have tried to make it, this asana routine can

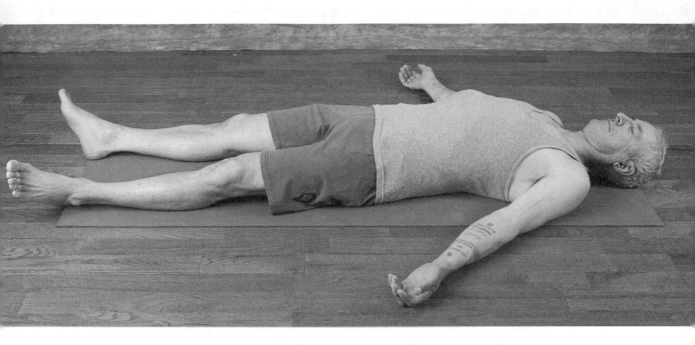

still be a fairly challenging practice. Step by step, one day at a time, it gets easier, and you will notice yourself changing—for the better.

FIGURE 6.17 Relaxation Posture

CHAPTER 7

CONNECT BODY AND MIND

CONSCIOUS BREATHING

Since you have been doing the ujjayi pranayama technique for quite a while now, it has perhaps become so familiar that you would benefit from a more in depth exploration of it. Let's go back to our explanation of pranayama from chapter 2 and review what the word means. If you remember, pranayama is comprised of two root words—*prana* and *yama*—which mean roughly "energy" and "control or restraint." So let's say that *pranayama* means "energy control" and is the practice of conscious breathing techniques. I prefer to call it "energy management." When we practice pranayama by controlling our breathing, we are actually learning to control and manage our *prana*, or our energy— both our intake and our expenditure. How can we relate this to what we have been doing so far?

WHERE ATTENTION GOES, PRANA FOLLOWS

One of the ways that prana enters the body is via the breath. The conscious breathing techniques of pranayama practices train us to maximize and increase our energy reserves. Focusing on the breath and consciously breathing require that your mind be here, in the moment. As a result, you will notice that you can actually have some control over what the mind is doing. Just as in asana, you will know when you are pushing too hard or relaxing too much. You can dial it up or down—you are in control of your energy. This is training. You are learning to use your energy effectively and in a sustainable way, and you will begin to see that when you are focused on your breath, your mind quiets down, the nervous system unwinds, the relaxation response kicks in, and eventually the symptoms of PTS and other anxiety disorders begin to soften and dissolve. The practice teaches you to pay attention to the movement of prana within yourself and how to use it. Just as important, it can also show you how you lose it.

Where attention goes, prana follows. This means that whatever we are thinking about draws our attention to that experience and creates an expenditure of energy. When we are plugged into a past traumatic event, for example a simple argument with a family member, just thinking about it takes energy. The less control we have over when and how we think about it, the more energy it drains from us, until we don't have a whole lot left to get through the day. Can you feel that when your mind is racing out of control and your body is tight as a drum, you are wasting energy? After an episode that triggers a flashback, for example, do you usually feel pretty depleted? It is exhausting—that is what I mean by expenditure of energy. Practicing pranayama trains us, as asana has already begun to do, to be aware of how we are allowing our energy to be washed away.

HOW PRANAYAMA BUILDS ON
YOUR ASANA PRACTICE

How does this prana that we are working to bring into the body travel around through the body? According to yoga theory, prana travels on *nadis,* or "tracks" in the "energy body," which is thought to be a field of energy surrounding and intersecting with our physical body. Our asana practice purifies and polishes these tracks and prepares us for pranayama—which is basically the practice of running prana "trains" down the nadi "tracks!" Once we have cleaned the tracks, repaired any broken tracks, and polished off the rust and dirt through our asana practice, then the prana can run smoothly and do its job of healing, balancing, energizing, and calming.

Probably the most important thing to say about the practice of pranayama (and this applies to any practice you might ever do, not just the practices that follow here) is that it should *never* upset you in any way—not physically, like causing you to be out of breath, or psychologically, like causing you to feel anxious or panicky. If at anytime you start to feel even the slightest bit uncomfortable, just calmly drop the practice and return to even, regular, natural breath.

BURNING OUT SAMSKARAS TO
REMOVE INNER OBSTACLES

In yoga practice, pranayama (like asana) is thought to be an important form of tapas, which you may remember means "to heat or burn." Continuing the work of asana, these pranayama practices help release toxins and blocks, burn impurities, and remove any obstacles in your storage reservoirs, making more room for prana. Mentally, they help to dig out old traumas and impressions and tendencies. So hang in here with me now because this is pretty far out *and* really fascinating.

In yoga philosophy, it is thought that all our daily experiences leave an indelible imprint on our subconscious, whether these experiences are conscious or unconscious, desirable or undesirable. These imprints are called *samskaras,* and they are thought to determine the moment-to-moment choices we make as well as the course of our lives. I imagine them like thumbprints on a pane of glass—imprints, impressions. We are creating these tracks every moment, with every action and thought. They are the energetic imprints of all our experiences and, according to yoga philosophy, they get stored in concentric layers of subtle energy fields that wrap around the body. Really! So the old stored memories of traumatic experiences you may have had as a warrior in battle, the ones that may be causing your insomnia, anger, anxiety, or any post-traumatic stress, are literally still imprinted in your unconscious or subconscious mind. Any flashbacks you may have aren't your imagination, and they aren't coming out of nowhere. And what we are learning now is that mind-body practices, like pranayama, can help to clean the glass, so to speak, and wipe away these old impressions—just burn them out of our energy fields so they no longer have the potential to activate and burst into the conscious mind—pretty powerful and worth a shot at trying them.

As we learn and practice these techniques, going from the simple to the more complex, we learn to pay closer and closer attention to what we are doing. The following practices help us to develop the intensity and the ability (as I keep saying over and over) to *be here right now.* They pull us back from our mental wanderings to being with what actually is. The ultimate purpose of pranayama is to control the movement of the mind. We learn that every moment, every second, we have a choice, a choice to be here or to spin off into some old movie or fearful memory. Yoga tells us: Practice being here. It's good for you. It will quiet your mind. When your mind is quiet for a long enough period of time, you will have glimpses of your True Self. You will like these glimpses. You will want to see more. You will have more available prana. You will have greater access to your power. You will feel more peaceful, happier, more content with life.

PREPARATION FOR PRANAYAMA PRACTICE

Practicing pranayama is not a walk in the park. It requires attention, a desire to learn the practice, and commitment to *practice* the practice. Here are the general instructions to be aware of as you engage this path.

Time of Day

Morning practice is a great way to wake yourself up for the day. Evening practice is excellent preparation for sleep. It quiets the mind and relaxes the nervous system. However, you want to allow at least two or three hours after you have eaten dinner before you do your evening pranayama. And it's not recommended to practice after a big meal or after a couple of beers or glasses of wine. Of course, you *can,* but it won't be particularly effective.

Posture Basics

Pranayama is done with the eyes closed, in a comfortable seated position. You may sit on the floor or in a chair. If you are ill or injured, you may do these exercises lying down.

Develop Your Practice Slowly

When you begin pranayama practice, start with the basics and work slowly and mindfully over time to develop mastery of the breath. You cannot be in a hurry. I know I've said this a dozen times already, but I can't repeat it enough: The most important aspect of this training, like your work in asana, is to develop the ability to focus your attention on one thing over an ever increasing length of time. Pranayama is not an exercise to develop lung capacity. That will happen as a result of years of practice, but it is not the actual objective.

Signs to Ease Off the Practice or Readjust It

As you learn and practice any, or all, of the three pranayama techniques that follow, keep in mind that doing pranayama should never disturb you in any way. It is important for me to say again that it should not disturb the evenness of your breath, nor your balance—psychological and physiological—nor your sense of well-being. During the practice, you should not feel any pressure inside your eyes or ears. If you feel any nausea, light-headedness or dizziness, you are either straining or doing too much, and you need to back off and return to a more preliminary practice. If you force the breath or strain or struggle with it in any way, you will stress both your lungs and your mind. Some relaxed effort is necessary to focus the mind, but it should not cause agitation or anxiety.

By engaging in any of the many pranayama techniques available to yoga practitioners, you may elevate or lower your energy level, depending on your needs. In either case, the result should be calmness and clarity. If you are tired or feel depleted, and you are doing pranayama to increase your vitality, it will not make you hyperactive or nervous if done correctly. Doing pranayama to increase energy is *not* like drinking a cup of coffee. The practice strengthens and soothes the nervous system, enabling the entire structure to function more effectively. It does not artificially stimulate the nervous system as caffeine does.

If, on the other hand, you are doing pranayama to relax, you can use it during the day to chill out, to bring your nervous system into a more tranquil state, and at night to help prepare for sleep. In this case, it is *not* like taking an antidepressant, anti-anxiety medication, or a sleeping pill. It is a natural, organic method to return your body to an effortless rhythm of balance between expanding and contracting, waking and sleeping, working and resting, outputting and recharging.

Using the Bandhas

To keep the prana traveling on the tracks, we need to have a *closed system* so that no prana will leak out. What keeps the prana traveling in the system is the use of our old friends, the locks.

You have already begun to learn and practice the locks, or the bandhas, in your asana practice. Now you will continue to use both locks—mula bandha and uddiyana bandha—throughout the pranayama practice, as best you can. Be relaxed about it. Think of these two locks as energetic "upliftments." Imagine that you can keep them in place with just a little attention. When we give a little attention to pulling up in these two areas, that "pulling up" intention is what is meant by "lock." This lifting up action helps to support our practice—whether asana or pranayama—and it fuels the agni (the fire) that we want to create through our practice to burn impurities and work out those samskaras, or the traumas and anxieties.

To do this, just make it your *intention* to give some *attention* to keeping the locks *locked*. I like to imagine that I am posting a sentry at a gate at the base of the spine (at the perineum) and another at a gate at the navel center just below the belly button, where these two bandhas are centered. Let those two sentries be sure to keep the two gates locked. If the locks are allowed to open during your pranayama practice, energy will leak out, which isn't a totally awful thing, as it is going to take us awhile to be able to keep these bandhas in place anyway. But we want to work toward a sustainable, *closed system,* so that eventually we can blast the prana around the body and blow out anything that disrupts the field.

Transitioning Out of the Practice

For all three practices, the best way to transition from being *in* the practice to being *finished* is to slowly allow your natural breath to return. Sit quietly for a few moments, keeping your eyes closed. Open your eyes slowly and return gently to the outside world.

OVERVIEW OF PRANAYAMA PRACTICE

You can practice first thing in the morning to help get your day started, last thing at night to help you relax and prepare for sleep, and anytime to deal with stress, fatigue, or anxiety.

I have used the Sanskrit names for each of these breathing techniques. They might be confusing to you at first, but I have defined each of them and have tried to be consistent in their usage. I thought you would enjoy knowing their proper names.

1. Warm up with three-part yoga breathing awareness.

2. Continue with the three pranayama techniques:

    - *Sama vritti ujjayi* breathing, which simply means "equal" (*sama*) "movement" (*vritti*) "of the breath" (*ujjayi*): in other words, focusing your attention on balancing the inhalation and the exhalation

    - *Langhana* and *brahmana,* lengthening the exhalation and the inhalation

    - *Nadi shodana,* alternate nostril breathing

Preliminary Exercise
Three-Part Yoga Breathing Awareness

Before you begin any of the pranayama techniques that follow, first spend time with this preliminary exercise: three-part yoga breathing. If you can, do it a few times a day for a few weeks, maybe up to a month or so. This can serve as a short introduction to pranayama as a stand-alone practice, or it can be continued for longer periods of time as a relaxation and stress-management practice. It is a very handy practice to carry around in your back pocket and whip out whenever you feel like you are getting close to the edge.

This simple preliminary routine will help you to familiarize yourself with your natural breath and the depth and capacity of your breathing pattern. That way, when you begin to practice the actual pranayama techniques, you will have a solid and correct foundation upon which to build your practice.

This should take you at least five to seven minutes.

1. Sit on the floor with your legs crossed, or in a chair with your back supported and feet flat on the floor. Close your eyes. Feel the weight of your body seated wherever you are. Pretend you are a big, old majestic tree. Imagine that you are "grounding down" or setting roots deep into the earth. Feel your connection to the earth. Let that feel good for you—like you are being supported and protected by the earth. Notice that you are breathing. Try not to change your breath. Just watch it. As you breathe in and out of the nose, feel the natural rhythm of your breath as you inhale and exhale.

2. Bring your awareness to your lower belly, below your navel. Feel the belly as it expands on the inhalation

as the breath moves into the lower part of your lungs, and then contracts, or returns to rest on the exhalation. Repeat this for at least five breath cycles.

3. Now move your awareness up slightly above your navel to the solar plexus. See if you can have awareness of your diaphragm (the big, dome-shaped respiratory muscle at the solar plexus) contracting and descending—expanding the abdomen on your inhalation, and then relaxing and rising—returning to a resting position on your exhalation. See if you can feel your rib cage expanding and contracting as you breathe. Do this for at least five breath cycles.

4. Finally, move your awareness to your upper chest and feel how it subtly expands on your inhale and contracts on your exhale. See if you can feel the awareness of your breath all the way up to the collarbone. Do this for five breath cycles.

5. Now you will put these three elements together. Instead of simply watching the natural breath come in and out, you will begin to control it a little bit as you move into the three-part yogic breath. This time on one inhalation, starting at the bottom as you begin inhaling, feel the first one-third of your inhalation in your low belly, then feel the next third of your breath in the middle—just above the waist and in the ribcage—and finally, fill the lungs all the way up to the collarbone. At first, you might feel like you aren't having much success—this is normal. Stay with it and just *imagine* as you are moving your attention from your belly to your rib cage to your chest. Like anything, the more you practice, the easier this gets.

6. Then reverse that awareness and empty the lungs in the opposite order—exhaling at the top third, then the middle third, and lastly, the bottom section, feeling the movement from the chest down to the middle of the rib cage, and finally down to the belly.

7. Continue to move back and forth, not forcing or straining, not breathing too slowly or too quickly. Inhale and breathe into the belly, then the ribs, and then the chest. Then exhale and empty the chest, the ribs, and the belly. Go on in this way for several minutes, perhaps taking fifteen to twenty more breaths.

8. To end, bring your awareness back to the natural movement of your breath as you inhale and exhale. Relax any effort and relinquish any control over the breath. Notice the overall expansion and contraction of your torso as you breathe. Let the breath be natural and relaxed. Take several breaths. I like to sit for a bit before I open my eyes, then rub my hands together for a moment or two, and then rest my eyes in the palms of my hands, slowly opening my eyes. Sit quietly and take the time to notice how you feel.

Pranayama Practice 1 Sama Vritti
Ujjayi (Equal Movement Victorious Breathing)

Sama vritti ujjayi pranayama is a powerful balancing and centering technique. It uses the same ujjayi breathing that you first learned in chapter 2 and that you continued to use in your asana practice. Now we will take it to a new level and use it in a slightly different way—as a stand-alone practice to get energized and focused for the day, to relax and center, or to slow down and unwind before bed.

The Sanskrit words *sama vritti* mean "equal movement," and when referring to the breath, the idea is to make the inhalation and the exhalation exactly equal in length. The technique of taking an existing practice and refining it to a point that requires greater attention is one of the brilliant ways this yoga methodology grabs us and takes us deeper into ourselves.

Getting Started

1. Sit quietly, ideally in a place where you won't be interrupted. Sit on the floor or in a chair with your feet on the floor. If you are injured or ill or unable to sit for any reason, do the practice lying down.

    Close your eyes. Take a moment to notice what is going on around you. Listen. What do you hear? Take interest. Scan your external environment. Notice what sounds you hear.

    As a military man or woman, isn't this what you have already been trained to do? Pay attention. So for now, just listen. It's okay. You're okay. Just breathe.

    Bill Bradley, an American hall of fame basketball player and a former three-term Democratic US senator, used to talk about developing a "sense of where you are" on the basketball court. For him, it was an amazing ability to sense what was going on 360 degrees around him. This is certainly a skill that you can totally relate to and that you most likely have developed to a pretty advanced degree. If you think about it objectively, it is a pretty cool skill to have. Remind yourself that, even if you are struggling with hyperarousal and jumping out of your skin every time a car backfires or a plane flies overhead, it isn't all bad. Think of all the situations when it is nice to be fully awake and aware, when what you learned and experienced in the military comes in handy.

In fact your yoga training is teaching you to be more *awake, conscious,* and *sensitive* to what is going on, not only around you, but also inside of you. So this isn't about trying to dumb down your senses and turn you into a no-feeling, no-sensing zombie, which makes the practice a huge advantage over some drugs! Rather, it is about learning to make friends with our awareness, and to then tame it, train it, control it, and direct it.

2. After a few moments, turn your attention inward and scan your internal environment. This will require a bit of a shift. Stick with it. What is going on inside? Focus in on the various systems of the body, one at a time: circulation, digestion, elimination, and the nervous systems. Take the time to actually *look* at them. See what is going on. How does your belly feel? Okay today? Or a little queasy? Don't rush through this. Focus. What about your stomach? Your heart? Racing or calm and steady? Learn to notice this stuff. Where do you notice tightness or compression or upset? Conversely, where do you notice smooth, calm operation? Finally bring your attention to your respiration, your breathing. Watch your natural breath for a moment or two. Observe the rhythm.

The Practice

1. Slowly engage the throat contraction that creates the ujjayi sound (as explained in chapter 2) and continue to breathe, only now with ujjayi in place. Take ten or fifteen full ujjayi breaths. Establish a rhythm and follow the breath with your attention.

2. Count out your inhalation and your exhalation. In other words, as you breathe in, count "one, two, three" and so forth, until you have finished the inhalation. Then exhale and count out the length of that breath. Let's say to begin, you find that you are breathing in to the count of three and out to the count of four. The ratio is three to four. Or your inhalation and exhalation may be the same length. Just watch and see what you observe. Don't change it yet. Just observe what is happening at the moment.

3. Slowly continue to breathe, counting the length of both the inhalation and the exhalation. You might want to find a point in your body where you can feel the breath, maybe the belly or the heart center at the middle of the chest. Choose one point along the breath's path and watch over it. Hold your attention there as if you were guarding the breath. Guard the breath for a few minutes, a few times a day for a few weeks, or whatever it takes for you to get comfortable.

4. Once you are guarding the breath easily, put the sama vritti, the equal movement part of the technique in place—balance the inhalation and exhalation, making them equal in length. So now your count for the in-breath and the out-breath becomes the same. Instead of three to four, perhaps the ratio is now three to three, or four to four. This might already be happening naturally, or perhaps you will need to adjust your breath slightly. Pay attention and find the balance between the inhalation and the exhalation until they are equal. Do this for ten or fifteen breaths.

5. Once you feel comfortable, drop the counting and just focus on keeping the two halves equal without counting. This is true spontaneous sama vritti. At this point, you will probably be breathing more slowly and deeply, perhaps taking six or seven breaths per minute, maybe fewer. Work with this pranayama practice for five minutes, which means you will take around thirty or thirty-five breaths. Nice. You might want to set a timer before you start. After you can do five minutes pretty easily, increase to ten minutes next time.

6. Once your time is up, slowly drop the ujjayi breathing and return to natural breath. Watch your natural breath for a moment or two. See if you notice any change in your natural breath from when you started.

7. Keeping your eyes closed, twist slowly while you are seated, first to the right, then to the left. Then arch backward, with your hands on the floor behind you (if you are sitting on the floor), and extend the spine. Then round forward with your hands on the floor in front of you and flex the spine. Rub your hands together, and then rest the palms of your hands over your eyes. Slowly open your eyes and release your hands. Smile.

Final Note

When you sit and try to practice this on your own, it might not be so easy for you. You might get bored after a day or two and wonder what comes next. You might think, *Well, maybe whatever comes next will be less boring.* Forget about it. Stay focused.

Possibly, you will be interrupted by a sensation in your body or by a sound or by thoughts that pop up out of nowhere—thoughts you would prefer not to have. This is totally normal and happens to everyone. It is going to happen and it's okay. The best attitude to have is to just shrug your shoulders, notice the distraction, and say, "Oh, well," and keep going. Things are going to distract you—over and over. But with practice it will happen less and less. You *will* get better at this.

It is fine to go on and read through all three of the pranayama practices, just to have a sense of where you are going with all this. Then you will need to come back to the first practice, start at the beginning, and work through the others one at a time.

Pranayama Practice 2 Langhana and Brahmana (Exhale and Inhale Extension)

This is a two-part pranayama practice that focuses on lengthening the breath—both the in-breath and the out-breath. The first part of the practice focuses on extending the exhalation and is called *langhana,* which means to "contract or reduce." Langhana pranayama refers to a drawing out or a lengthening of the out-breath. The second part focuses on extending the inhalation and is called *brahmana,* which means "vast expanse" or "to grow, expand." Brahmana pranayama refers to the lengthening of the in-breath. These two different pranayama techniques each have a different physiological and psychological effect as a result of the opposing aspects of the two different energies each carries.

Extending the exhalation is thought in yoga philosophy to be a *contracting* or *calming* force that reduces and purifies. Exhalation is also the part of the breath cycle that activates the *parasympathetic* portion of the autonomic nervous system. When we want to help a friend relax, what do we say? "Take a breath." What do they do? They take a big breath, and then slowly, and usually extendedly, they exhale! A big *sigh!* It is instantaneously relaxing.

Extending the inhalation, on the other hand, is the opposite: an *expanding* or *energizing* force that nourishes and builds up. When we are startled, what do we do? We gasp. We inhale and grab a breath. This activates the *sympathetic* side of the autonomic nervous system. It is instantly activating.

So the effect of almost any exhalation (langhana) practice is to reduce, quiet, slow down, and calm. The effect of all inhalation (brahmana) practices is to expand, energize, and empower.

We begin with exhale-lengthening and focus pretty much exclusively on that because we want to purify and calm the body and mind before we begin to energize it and build it up. Also, it is more than likely that you are looking for a way to ramp down anxiety and tension. So it is quite possible that you may never get around to the inhale-lengthening portion of this practice. You might not need it. All you want is to begin to get control over the startle response, or over the sense of alienation you feel from your civilian friends and family, or over the tendency to avoid everything and everyone, including yourself. Exhaling helps us to get grounded, get anchored in our bodies, and settle into the present moment.

Having said that, it is important to realize that both practices can be beneficial and balancing. *Balancing* is the key word here. It isn't as if breathing in is bad and breathing out is good. It's about finding balance. Both portions of the breath cycle are essential for life and equally sacred.

What is more important is to learn to *notice* how you feel and identify what practice can help you in any given moment of the day. If you feel like you are on the edge with yourself, your kids, your partner or spouse, your superiors or peers, and are about to jump out of your skin with anxiety, impatience, aggravation, and the like, or want help in falling asleep, do exhale lengthening! If, however, you are lethargic, depressed, tired, sleep deprived and needing to stay awake, or listless, then do inhale lengthening.

The Langhana Practice (Lengthening the Exhalation)

1. Just as you did for the previous pranayama practice, take a few minutes to settle and switch to listening and attending mode. Sit comfortably. Settle. Scan the external environment. Scan the internal environment. Bring your attention to your natural breath.

2. Engage the bandhas. This might simply mean visualizing a small beam of light and "posting light sentries" at the points of mula bandha (the perineum, or floor, of the pelvis) and uddiyana bandha (a few inches below the navel) and asking the sentries to keep the "gates locked." That can be enough. Every once in a while, just check in with your sentries and make sure they are still on the job—keeping anyone or anything from "going out" of those gates. It's like keeping the FOB secure and the wire intact. This awareness keeps the energy in and moving up. Good.

3. Begin pranayama practice 1, sama vritti ujjayi pranayama, the technique in which you maintain equal movement, or uniform length of the inhalation and the exhalation. Let the ujjayi breath be very gentle and barely audible. It will sound a little different and a little quieter than it does in your asana practice or even than it does in the preceding pranayama where you use the ujjayi breathing as a stand-alone practice. When lengthening the exhalation and

inhalation, the throat contraction will still be in place, but the sound will be very soft and barely audible.

4. Gradually begin to lengthen your exhale. For example, if you have been breathing in and out to a count of four for the sama vritti, now try to exhale a bit more, perhaps to a count of five or six for a four-to-five or four-to-six ratio between inhalation and exhalation. Find a count that is comfortable, settle on that, and stick with it. Remember, the effect here is to slow down and quiet the nervous system. According to yoga philosophy, langhana supports elimination and has a cleansing and restorative effect on all the organs, especially those in the abdominal region. See if you can sit long enough and pay close enough attention so that you feel the calming effect and the slowing down.

5. As you exhale, imagine you are releasing blocks and impurities in the lower belly. As you extend the exhalation, you are using the easy energetic lift of the bandhas to squeeze negative impressions out of your body and psyche. Focus on the lower abdominal region. Don't force or strain. Don't be mad. Just push out what prevents you from experiencing peace of mind and equipoise. Use your locks to help move impurities up and out.

    Here's a visualization that can help with this. In yoga philosophy, the locks are thought to help bring up the toxic elements in your mind and body to the solar plexus, the "fire center." This center is called the *manipura,* which means "palace of jewels." Here, energetic diamonds and emeralds and rubies are thought to burn with such a brilliant light that they eliminate toxins. Hopefully that is a beautiful visualization for you—to think that deep in the center of your body, you have a bright and magnificent treasure trove. Here, the ancient yoga texts say, impurities are burned and reduced to their fundamental chemical makeup of atoms of carbon, hydrogen, nitrogen, and oxygen. Then they are returned to the "source" or just sent out into the world as neutral energy. Nice thought, isn't it? We wouldn't want to give our personal toxins to anyone else.

6. Be sure you are inhaling naturally. If you have to gasp for breath, you've pushed way too hard on the exhalation or it has gone on too long. If you exhale for too long, the inhalation becomes short and fast, and you will find yourself gulping for air. In no way should the breath extensions disturb a comfortable, natural rhythm of the breath, or bother you in any way.

7. Keep going. Again, exhale and lengthen. Use the first few breaths to actively detoxify your cells and tissues. It's like you're dumping out the trash. Then settle and focus on a steady, rhythmic lengthening of the exhalation. With this method, you are emptying before trying to fill.

8. Do two rounds of twelve breaths each. When that becomes relaxed and unhurried, do two rounds of twenty-four breaths each. Take several weeks to just practice with the exhalation.

9. Once that is easy, further extend the exhalation. If you are still breathing in to a count of four, for example, see if you can breathe out to a count of six or seven, or not quite twice the length of the

inhalation, a ratio of four to six, or two to three. Remember, if the rhythm of the inhalation is disturbed in any way by the exhalation, then shorten the duration of the exhalation again, until the rhythm of the complete cycle is smooth and natural.

10. Now that you have created some space in your energy body through the removal of obstacles and impressions, if you feel as if you would like to go on and learn the inhale-lengthening portion of this practice, you can continue to the second part of this pranayama practice. However, if you feel that you are still working primarily on ramping things down, getting grounded, trying to sleep, getting control of your explosive emotions, or connecting with self, family, and friends, then I recommend you skip the inhale-lengthening practice and go on to pranayama practice 3, nadi shodana.

The Brahmana Practice (Lengthening the Inhalation)

Once lengthening the exhalation becomes easy and comfortable, with no disturbances in the breath, you can begin to practice extending the inhalation.

1. Start in the same way as you did the langhana practice. Observe the breath's natural rhythm and begin to follow it. Engage the locks and begin ujjayi breathing. Continue as you started for the previous practice by keeping the inhalation and exhalation equal in duration.

2. Now begin to lengthen the inhalation. This is the practice of brahmana, of "expanding" or "growing" the inhalation somewhat, by a beat of one, two, or whatever is comfortable for you. If you are exhaling to a count of four, see if you can inhale to a count of

five or six. The ratio of inhalation to exhalation will then be six to four, or we could say three to two.

3. Exhale naturally. If the exhalation "pops" out or is even mildly explosive sounding, you have extended the inhalation too long. You need to recalculate and just practice extending the inhalation a little bit, by a count of one or two.

4. Keep the focus on the inhalation and its extension. It might take a little extra attention to switch over to focusing on the inhalation after your previous focus on the exhalation. You might find yourself slipping back into the now almost automatic practice of exhalation extension. This is okay. Just pay attention and take this one breath at a time. It's all good training.

5. Remember to keep your sentries posted and the locks in place. They will support a *closed system* in your energy body so the prana can run at full power through the channels that carry it and empower and expand the energy body (and clear out the crap!). Focus on the chest and heart center. Do two rounds of twelve breaths each. When that becomes relaxed and unhurried, do two rounds of twenty-four breaths each. Take several weeks just to practice with extending the inhalation.

6. What do you notice? What happens during the extension of breath? What is the difference between the feelings you have when extending the inhalation versus the exhalation? As you observe these distinctions, you can start to use these practices at different times of the day and for different purposes, to energize or relax your state of being.

Pranayama Practice 3 Nadi Shodana
(Nerve Purification and Alternate Nostril Breathing)

The third method of pranayama we will work with in this chapter is called *nadi shodana,* literally "channel purification," a form of alternate nostril breathing. One nostril is alternately held closed while breathing occurs through the other. This is the most advanced of the three practices in this chapter.

This is a very powerful and effective practice for calming the mind and quieting the nervous system. It balances the right and left hemispheres of the brain as well as the parasympathetic and sympathetic nervous systems, so it has a very strong leveling effect that you can feel when you practice. It also evens out the relationship between the cooling and heating energies of the body, referred to in yoga as the *ida* and the *pingala,* or the feminine and masculine, the lunar and solar energies of the body. This is an adaptogenic practice, which means it will cool and calm you down if you are too agitated or stirred up. Conversely, if you are too cool or inactive, it will warm you up and energize you.

It might be a little difficult to get this whole process of regulating the breath through the nose going smoothly, but with practice it becomes easy. Some days the nasal passageways will be completely clear and open, and other days you might be a little stuffy.

Getting Started

1. You will use your right hand for nostril control. To do this, fold the index and middle fingers of your right hand down into your palm. Use your thumb to close the right nostril by placing your right thumb on

the right side of your nose, just below the nasal bone, where the nose becomes softer and turns to cartilage, and just above where the nostrils begin to flare.

To close the left nostril, use both your ring finger and little finger (if that isn't possible or feels uncomfortable, use your index finger to close the left). Place the ring and little finger (or index finger) on the left side of the nose in the same place as your thumb was placed on the right.

Even if it isn't possible for you to use your hands, you can still do this practice. Apply your attention, without the hands, to concentrate first on one nostril and then the other and just *imagine* that you are breathing through either the left or the right nostril. This is a very powerful way to do the practice, and I often use this technique when teaching nadi shodana pranayama to both advanced and beginning practitioners. It is a great way to demonstrate the power of our mind. Most people are really surprised when they discover that they feel they are actually able to do the practice without using their hands.

2. Unlike the two previous exercises, you will use ujjayi breathing only to begin the practice. After that you will control the breath with the diaphragm and in the nostril passageway rather than the throat. Before you start, get a sense of how this will feel. Apply pressure and close both nostrils. Now release one side and try breathing in and out through that nostril while holding the opposite nostril fully closed. Switch and try the other side. Blow your nose!

3. Take a moment to check in with the locks. As with the other pranayama practices, do your best

to keep the "upliftment" energy of the bandhas in place. Send your sentries to keep an eye on the energy centers and to keep the impurities moving up toward the fire center at the solar plexus.

The Practice

1. Close your eyes. Take three stabilizing ujjayi breaths through both nostrils, then prepare to move your right hand into place. Drop the ujjayi, and begin by closing the left nostril with your fourth and fifth (ring and little) fingers, and breathe in through the right nostril. Now close the right nostril with your thumb while still holding the left nostril closed, pause for a beat, and then release the left nostril and breath out through the left. This starts the first round. Start slowly and gently.

2. Pause for a second, then breathe back in through the left nostril while holding the right nostril closed. Then close the left nostril as well, holding both closed, pause, then open the right, breathe out again, and pause. This completes the round.

3. Do this again from right to left and back again. Close left, in right, close both, pause, out left, pause, in left, close both, pause, out right, pause. Do this a few times to get the hang of it.

4. Make sure you have completely dropped the ujjayi breath and are regulating the breath with the diaphragm and in the nostril canal. This might be hard to do at first, especially if you are used to ujjayi breathing.

5. Once you get a rhythm going, practice sama vritti (equal movement) of the breaths. Match the inhalation with the exhalation. Develop a baseline count, like "in two, three, four" and "out two, three, four." Don't rush the breath, but don't draw it out excessively or make it too slow, either. Find a moderate pace comfortable for you.

6. Once you feel comfortable with this technique and find your rhythm, you can begin to do a few more rounds. Work up to a set of twelve rounds. That will likely take you between three and four minutes. Once that becomes easy, do two or three sets of twelve rounds and work up to anywhere from six to twelve minutes.

7. To finish, as with all the pranayama practices, slowly return to the natural breath. Sit for a few moments with your eyes closed and notice how you feel. What changes do you experience in your natural breath or your system in general? How do you feel? Slowly open your eyes and take some time to return to normal activity. Notice how the world around you looks. People often report how clear and bright everything seems in the outside world, as if, while they had their eyes closed, there had been a rainstorm that washed everything clean.

LEARNING ACCEPTANCE

Our practice in a general sense—whether it is doing asana, pranayama, sitting and listening to the wind and rain, or peeling carrots—is about noticing when we become distracted from the present moment and our awareness of *now*. In a formal practice like asana or pranayama, it is noticing when we have been distracted from the specific object of our concentration. It is about noticing, not judging, just noticing every feeling, every thought, as it dawns and bubbles up, and then watching where that takes us. We are trying to see, ever more clearly, just what it is we actually do with our prana. We come to realize that we don't just expend energy by running, raking leaves, driving to work, or cooking dinner, but that we also mentally expend tons of energy by unconsciously allowing our minds to wander off to other people, places, and times. It can take awhile to actually see these comings and goings, but it is through our practice that we begin to develop this objectivity.

What is this noise? Where *are* all these seemingly out of nowhere, random, out-of-control, stressed-out thoughts coming from? Where are they stored? Where do we go when we start this thinking business? Memories emerge from the depths of our past experiences, and fears about what will happen to us loom in our brains. How will we manage? We think about things we should be doing, or friends we need to call, or family members we saw last week or last year. If we have had a fight or upsetting interaction with someone, or someone has criticized us, thoughts of that pop up, and we begin to mutter and grumble. We "send our spirit on negative missions," as medical intuitive Carolyn Myss so aptly describes the process. Our inner dialogue lays out a world where we get even or make ourselves more comfortable, or even less comfortable. We are very busy trying to rearrange reality to be more suitable to our needs. But the reality is whatever is happening *now*. Perhaps we are just mildly anxious or stressed out. Or perhaps we are having a serious panic attack. We have to start where we are.

In the case of almost any anxiety disorder, like PTS, the reality is that our brain can really spin out of control. We may want to put down the memories of past traumatic events, for example, but can't quite figure out how. And in the case of catastrophic, traumatic events, they seem to have a life of their own—they take our attention, our energy. They pop up in the middle of the night. They are triggered by the most benign events. And there we go again, spinning off and trying to function under the weight of the negative physiological and psychological effects that our mind is causing for our body.

According to yoga, the world is exactly as it needs to be, and everything that happens to us is exactly what needs to be happening at every moment—whether we like it or not, whether it is comfortable or not, whether it is pleasurable or painful. The whole point of our practice, and of using yoga to heal and regain our lives, is to try to train ourselves to hang out in the present as much as possible, no matter what is going on, to *accept what is.* And that point of view is hell to accept when you are suffering! It seems like complete bullshit, I know.

But we have to look at this in a balanced way. Again, I ask, "What is the option?" We can whine and moan and say, "Oh, this isn't fair. This shouldn't be happening to me," and on and on. But the reality is that it *is* happening. Accepting *what is* doesn't mean we tolerate endless suffering. And it doesn't mean that if a past traumatic memory keeps popping up that we just allow it to consume us and go on, and on, and on. It means, first, we accept it and notice it. We don't stuff it back down because it is painful. We accept things only a *moment* at a time. We sit back, at a safe distance, and objectively watch it. Second, we remind ourselves that now, in this present moment, things are relatively predictable, we are out of harm's way, we are in *control,* and we have tools that offer support. We can safely allow that memory to surface, pass through us, and be vaporized back into minute, neutral subatomic particles that dissipate into space.

Our asana practice has begun to train us to be present and accept this moment, and that is what pranayama continues to train us to do. Both practices give us tools that help us to deal with painful experiences—whether past or present—in a protected way. That is the crux of all our work, and that is all there is—to be *here* whether we are sick or healthy, happy or miserable, clear or confused. It is through developing this awareness that we start to notice how the chaotic and random noise in our head actually begins to quiet down. The more we can do that, the more we move toward health, happiness, and clarity—toward freedom.

CHAPTER 8

TURN INWARD

THE PRACTICE OF YOGA NIDRA, OR CONSCIOUS SLEEP

When you live with the day-to-day threat of direct combat, as warriors do when they're deployed, you accumulate tension, a lot of tension. If you are an infantry warrior operating in hostile territory 24/7, your experience will most likely be different from that of someone who is in a support role, operating inside the wire at the FOB. Although danger can be delivered in different ways, it still creates constant stress, which can be substantial—whether it is the stress of constant ambushes and firefights or the stress of random mortar attacks.

Although people who have not served in the military may not understand what it means to be a warrior, we can all relate to the accumulation of tension. No matter who we are, we accumulate tension—not just warriors, but families of deployed service men and women, veterans, civilians, everyone. Whether we work like banshees or sit on the couch all day, whether we think too much or not enough, sleep or don't sleep, whether we are kind or total SOBs—tension gathers, like dust, in every nook and cranny of the body's physical, mental, emotional, and psychic sheaths.

We all experience tension, and we know how tension seems to gather force as it festers in our body or mind. If we have a stressful thought or a flashback, our stomach gets tense, then our head, then our neck and shoulders, and then every other system in the body. It's not as if the rest of the body is clueless about what is going on. First we are tense, then grumpy, then perhaps depressed, then angry, then exhausted. The progression might be different for different individuals, but you get the point. The symptoms are mild at first: irritability, indigestion, irritable bowel syndrome, heartburn, headache, stiff neck and muscles, insomnia, and so on. But left ignored, any of these warning signs can lead to collective psychological distress, dis-ease, and all kinds of chaos and disorder in our professional, family, and social life. Either we *do something about it,* or eventually we deal with more serious illnesses and issues.

RELAXATION: THE FIRST STEP

While the path of yoga addresses a whole lot more than simply creating relaxation, relaxation is the first step. If we want a more peaceful world, we have to learn how to relax and join our own body and mind in synchronicity. Everything you have been working on up until now in your practice—the third limb of asana, the fourth limb of pranayama through the breath work—has been essentially, "doing something about it!" All of the elements you are learning have come together to help you begin to alleviate tension and stress, and let go and relax. By training yourself to pay attention to the present moment through anchoring your attention to your movements and breathing, you are minimizing the seemingly uncontrollable, random wanderings of the mind, which, as you well know, can recreate unpleasant or stressful memories, or can jump ahead to worries about the future.

CONSCIOUS SLEEPING

You have done a good deal of preparatory work that could be compared to digging up earth and taking out weeds to prepare for a garden plot. Now we'll move into working with a powerful practice that will plant some seeds. This is an effective technique that both active duty and veteran military service men and women will appreciate having in their tool kit. I have taught this not only to warriors, but also to people in all walks of life, and everyone loves this practice of yoga nidra.

The word *nidra* means "sleep," which is, ironically, not something we would ordinarily associate with yoga. We want to be conscious, aware, and not asleep when we do yoga. So why in the world would we want to do yoga nidra? When the word *nidra* is paired with the word *yoga,* as in *yoga nidra,* it means something a little different than just sleep. It means "sleep with a trace of awareness." It is a guided practice of meditation, really, where you are lying down, motionless, and led into a very deeply relaxed state. It is a state of mind between wakefulness and dream sleep where the mind quiets down to the point where you are just about to fall asleep, but you don't fall asleep. You maintain a link to consciousness. Maybe it sounds a little scary, but as my friend and student Suzanne Manafort, who directs the Mindful Yoga Therapy for Veterans project, says, "It is nothing creepy," and it's completely safe.

Yoga nidra is a way to experience the fifth limb of yoga: pratyahara. *Pratyahara* means "withdrawal" and refers to any practice that "pulls in" our senses. Instead of being drawn out and absorbed by the sights and sounds and smells of the world around us, or the memories fed to us by our thoughts, the senses look and listen inward and are used to explore the inner world of the present moment. It is really a remarkable experience, and once you are in an environment where you can feel safe and in control, you will find you are able to let go and settle into a deeply peaceful state of mind. It is a completely voluntary process and does not lead to diminished awareness, but to a super-aware, yet deeply peaceful, state of mind. What makes me think this is comforting, and perhaps even easy for a warrior, is that this skill of super-awareness has already been developed. It isn't that you want to eliminate awareness! That is exactly what we *are* trying to cultivate with yoga. The difference is that we want to be able to be in command of our awareness, *control* it, and use that ability with fine discernment.

SLOWING THE BRAIN WAVES

Yoga nidra can be thought of as a prelude to meditation. The practice will help to prepare you for the meditation techniques given in the next chapter. The process relaxes you. It is slightly hypnotic in the sense that, for most people, it guides the activity of the neurons of the brain to a slower frequency. This is the same thing that happens naturally when we fall asleep. The very moment of moving from being awake to being asleep can be precisely determined by physiological measurement of neuronal activity. The neurons are the brain cells and the very same guys we are trying to get to quiet down and stop the incessant mental noise they make when thinking is out of control. The brain really does slow down from the higher frequencies of thinking, for example, to the slower frequencies of sleep—whether light sleep, dream sleep, or deep sleep.

If you think of the exact moment when you fall asleep as a line drawn across a piece of paper, that line is called the *sleep threshold* (see figure 8.1). Just above the line we are still awake. Just below the line we have gone to sleep. All the various states of mental activity, whether thinking or sleeping, operate at different frequencies—the speed, or number of times per second, at which the neurons in the brain are firing, or going through their electro-chemical reactions to process information. When we are frantically worrying or thinking, it's like going at warp speed. When we are relaxed, just cruisin', not thinking frantically, the activity slows down. When we fall asleep, it slows way down. This process is controlled by the autonomic nervous system (ANS), which used to be called the *involuntary* nervous system, and which we first talked about in chapter 2.

But as I have mentioned previously, things like neurofeedback, also known as biofeedback, and meditation have shown us (and the world of medicine and science) that the processes controlled by the ANS are not so involuntary after all. As all of us who practice yoga experience, the mind can learn to control things like stress levels, respiration, heart rate, skin temperature, muscle tension, and brain wave activity. This is the level of control your yoga practice is slowly empowering you to have.

BRAIN WAVE ACTIVITY

AWAKE (conscious)	THINKING, DOING, TALKING	BETA WAVES (12–30 cycles/second)
	RELAXED, ALERT, NOT THINKING	ALPHA WAVES (8–12 cycles/second)
SLEEP THRESHOLD		
ASLEEP (unconscious) or YOGA NIDRA (conscious sleep)	DREAM SLEEP	THETA WAVES (4–7 cycles/second)
	DEEP SLEEP, NOT DREAMING	DELTA WAVES (1–4 cycles/second)

FIGURE 8.1. The state of yoga nidra (conscious sleeping) is a state of aware presence that can range from light to deep (7–1 cycles/second), depending on the experience of the practitioner.

When we enter the *state* of yoga nidra through the *process* of practicing yoga nidra, we are taking ourselves below the sleep threshold to the seven-cycles-per-second state of mind and lower, but we are not falling asleep.

In this way, yoga nidra is a state of mind between waking and dreaming. It is a practice that brings the deeper layers of our subconscious mind into conscious experience, and during which our consciousness travels through one layer of awareness to another, according to its capability and capacity. We actually tap into our subconscious mind—much like we dig a well to an underground aquifer to reach and pump up the water—and previously suppressed or buried material, which is the source of our psychological (and quite possibly) physiological pain, is brought up to the surface.

RELEASING TRAUMATIC SAMSKARAS (IMPRINTS)

When I travel, and my plane has to take off into thick cloud cover and flies into the gray cloak of complete opacity, I am always reminded of how deep-seated traumas and samskaras are released during yoga nidra. The total obscuring nature of the cloud cover is the perfect metaphor for how these suppressed memories or experiences are ultimately liberated.

When the plane takes off, you can see the ground for a while. Then the plane bumps around a little and ends up completely enveloped in clouds. It can be kind of a freaky situation. You *know* the ground is still down there, but you can't see it through the swath of gray. While you are *in* the clouds, you get bumped around—you don't know what is out there. But sooner or later, if you are climbing to 35,000 feet or so, you are going to rise high enough to see the clear, limitless horizon above the clouds. The samskaras that get released during yoga nidra do the same thing. As the memories and emotions come up from the dark recesses of our mind, they bump around, but they pass through the veil of obscurity and end up in the light.

When we are enveloped in the murkiness, it is hard to remember that the sun is still shining, waiting for us to come into the light again. But, as we gain altitude, we break through the clouds into clarity. In the light, in a safe and controlled setting, we can permit these samskaras to spontaneously rise to the surface. In this place of feeling good about ourselves, we can look at these images and past traumas, examine them, and allow then to harmlessly arise through the cloud cover and out into the vast emptiness of space, where they are neutralized and dissipated. Through the use of specific images and archetypes, used by the guide, these impressions can be liberated and harmlessly and painlessly dissolved.

RECASTING THE MIND

Unlike asana and pranayama practice, in yoga nidra it is not necessary to concentrate—in fact, you should not try to concentrate. You just keep your mind moving from point to point and, as you are guided through the process, allow yourself to dwell momentarily in the experience of the present. *Trying* to concentrate just ends up blocking the natural flow of consciousness as it spirals through deeper and deeper layers of awareness. If you just follow the instructions of your guide, you will find that you are able to deeply relax and open up your heart to new possibilities and visions. In the same way you melt iron and then cast it into the shape you wish to create, in yoga nidra, the mind can melt and be recast with good and creative impressions. It is an excellent practice to use if you are trying to remove a bad habit and replace it with a healthier one.

WHY DO YOGA NIDRA?

So why do we want to do this?

1. It is relaxing. It trains the body and mind to drop anxiety.

2. It puts us in a place where we are extending our conscious awareness a little deeper than just the state of being relaxed and awake (as you saw in figure 8.1). We aren't thinking, but we aren't asleep.

3. It puts us in a safe and receptive place where the thick, rusty, old buildup of *protective resistance* falls away and prana begins to flow in its place. The mind is melting, and we are open to positive and creative impressions.

4. It helps to open the subconscious and unconscious levels of the mind. (Yes, that is a good thing!) This helps us release deeply stored traumas, the samskaras, or imprints, that have been eating away at our health and well-being.

5. It can help us to sleep. If insomnia is an issue, this process can lead us to the sleep threshold and over into restful and restorative sleep.

6. It helps us prepare for meditation by further training the brain and making it possible for us to look deeper into the subconscious levels of our mind.

7. Research is beginning to validate that it can help to restore impaired biorhythms (the basic rhythms of life, like sleeping, eating, maintaining energy

levels). Disruption of these normal body rhythms can result in difficulty sleeping, forgetting to eat, feeling exhausted, mood swings, and so on.

PLANTING SEEDS BY SETTING AN INTENTION

Yoga nidra is a guided practice wherein the practitioner is led through the process by a teacher or by an audio recording. Instructions are given directly and simply, and there is a logical progression to the sequencing of directions. The instructor is only a guide. He or she simply delivers the technique. This is not persuasion or hypnosis or auto-suggestion. The student is learning to bring about his or her own state of relaxation by following the spoken instructions. That is why we have offered a guided audio recording that you can access by visiting SoundsTrue.com/YogaforWarriors/YogaNidra.

Yoga nidra is generally practiced lying down. The eyes are closed and the body is instructed to settle into stillness for the duration of the guided segment. The process of yoga nidra is generally divided into a number of segments. Like the many meditation techniques of different traditions, the techniques for teaching yoga nidra can vary slightly, but basically they follow a general format. There is the stage of preparation, then general physical relaxation, followed by the introduction of what is called in yoga *sankalpa,* or a "resolve" or "intention."

Having intention is thought to be one of the most important aspects of yoga nidra and a valuable means of training the mind. Yoga nidra is an extremely receptive state of consciousness, and the sankalpa is a short mental statement that we create for ourselves to heal an imbalance or to achieve a greater purpose in our life. It is impressed on our subconscious mind (by us) when it is sympathetic and sensitive to suggestion. The stating of our intention is like planting a seed deep in the subconscious. It will eventually sprout, grow, and burst forth, manifesting at the conscious level and bringing change in your life. No trauma or fear or habit is so deeply rooted that it cannot be changed.

Our intention should be a positive statement, and it should be directed at reaching the whole-life pattern, not only physically but also mentally, emotionally, and spiritually. We use it to help with our total transformation. It is stated simply, in the first-person, present tense, as if it were already occurring. Sometimes the idea for a sankalpa can pop nicely into our mind as we are moving into yoga nidra. Other times, it can set us off thinking, *Well, maybe this or maybe that,* trying to decide what the here-all, end-all, be-all *best* resolution might be. Uh, not a good idea. Give a little thought to what you are trying to work on in your life, before you start your yoga nidra practice. Maybe healing, maybe calming, maybe changing, whatever. Following are a couple of examples that might work for you, but feel free to create your own.

"My mind and body are in perfect synch."

"I trust the wisdom of my body."

"I am committed to living a life of perfect health."

"I am calm."

"I am rebuilding my life and moving toward greater light."

"I am healing and regaining health for the
benefit of all beings everywhere."

The setting of intention is generally followed by rotation of consciousness, body awareness, breathing, visualization, repetition of the intention, and finishing. This is a basic out-line of the way yoga nidra is most frequently taught.

INTEGRATING YOGA NIDRA: NO WORRIES

So at this point, you may be wondering when exactly you are supposed to *do* yoga nidra, and how you are going to fit it in with asana, pranayama practice, and the soon-to-come meditation practice. No worries. First of all, just go ahead and keep working your way through this entire book. Try all the practices—do each of them for a few days or weeks and see what you like and what works for you. Don't be in a hurry. Imagine you are on a long canoe trip, cruisin' down a gentle, slow-running stream or river in your part of the world. You paddle a little, pull into shore, hang out on the banks under overhanging trees. It is all quiet and peaceful. Birds sing. Maybe you see a moose, if you are in Vermont or Minnesota. Maybe you see a wolf or an eagle, if you are in Alaska. Breath by breath. Just easy. Try all the yoga practices.

I do think that it is important to do a little asana three to four days a week, at least. It helps you to get grounded and stable; it is great in general for strength, flexibility, balance, agility, and all around good health.

Whether you do yoga nidra or not, and especially if you do yoga nidra to help with insomnia, I happen to believe it is important to have a busy, daily program of asana and other physical exercise, like hiking or biking or swimming, or whatever works for you. Breathe. Get the body moving and keep it moving, so that when you rest, you *rest*, and it isn't a jittery, restless type of rest. It's real rest! I also think it is important to set aside a little time for a pranayama or meditation practice. Perhaps, five minutes of pranayama in the mornings to get you going—before work or before asana, maybe even before tea or coffee or teeth brushing. Then five to ten minutes of meditation in the evenings when things have quieted down.

Some people use yoga nidra regularly. Others respond better to doing langhana, or exhale-lengthening, before bedtime, or three-part yoga breathing. Some veterans prefer meditation. You will need to figure out for yourself what works and what doesn't work for you. I would definitely give this practice a try. You might want to use the audio that is offered online. Listen to it when you have time to lie down and relax for thirty or forty minutes, or when you *need* to relax. Before bed is good, but anytime is okay, if it helps you to ramp down an experience that is pushing the boundary of manageable.

Like asana and pranayama, the practice of yoga nidra will become a part of your yoga toolbox. It can now become one of several practices that you can use to help balance out your nervous system. It *is* a little different from some of the other yoga practices. Yoga nidra is a passive practice, one in which you are *led* through the process by an outside guide. It is not generally a practice that you would lead yourself through, although it can be done. Most of the warriors that either I, or some of my students work with, find it an incredibly helpful practice. I know many veteran and non-veteran yoga students who just *love* yoga nidra, and listen to a tape every night before going to bed, or in bed (after whatever it is they plan to do once they get to bed), to help put them to sleep. They may or may not fall asleep during the yoga nidra practice, but they find it much easier to sleep after the relaxation-inducing process of the practice.

When I can't sleep at night, I remember the techniques we do in meditation. If that doesn't work, I listen to a yoga nidra recording. It is the only thing I've found that really works. When I wake up, I feel rested instead of constantly groggy.
    LINE INFANTRY VETERAN, Operation Enduring Freedom

The Give Back Yoga Foundation offers a free Yoga Nidra CD or download to all veterans. See givebackyoga.org.

CHAPTER 9

THE PATH TO THE TRUE SELF

FINDING PEACE IN MEDITATION

The practice of yoga nidra has led us to this moment, and right into the sixth and seventh limbs of yoga: concentration and meditation, or as they are called in yoga, *dharana* and *dhyana*. This is special territory where we can really get to know ourselves and make friends with the One we meet. Just as we prepared for yoga nidra, our work has also been preparing us for this next step: meditation. Like the experience of yoga itself, meditation is what happens when we focus our attention on one thing and keep it connected to that one thing without distraction or interruption, whether it is the breath or a posture or a prayer or anything else. *Yoga,* or "union," is what happens when we can do that.

FROM CONCENTRATION TO MEDITATION

You can't learn to meditate until you learn to concentrate. Yoga tells us simply: "Learn to *concentrate* and it will lead you to meditation and a peaceful mind." There isn't a distinct border between concentration and meditation. One leads into the other, seamlessly over time and with practice. Technically, the *discontinuous* process we have been observing in our efforts to pay attention, of focusing, getting distracted, focusing, getting distracted, over and over again, is what is meant in yoga by *dharana,* or "concentration."

Concentration is a gathering in of our normally scattered energy. It is everything we have been doing in our practices until now to develop stability of the mind. So in training ourselves to concentrate, we are preparing for the meditation experience. Unlike dharana, *dhyana,* or "meditation," is a *continuous* connection between you and whatever it is you are meditating on, just like the flow of water pouring from a pitcher into a glass. It is an unbroken flow of awareness between two things.

This is what I love about the yoga methodology. It's not rocket science, but it *is* science, and it makes so much sense. It's a logical progression that we can follow rationally.

Our mind says to itself, *Hmm, first I learn to breathe and practice this breathing while I go through some exercises. Then I use the breathing alone to quiet the mind down and learn to be present without going through the physical routine. All of this is helping me to pay attention. Then, after a little practice in quieting the mind, I use yoga nidra to go a little deeper, and this prepares me for deeper concentration, which just means learning to notice—just as I have been doing—when I have been distracted from my point of focus, and then bringing my attention back, over and over again. This whole process leads me logically and clearly into meditation, which is what happens when I can stay focused on that one thing.*

Day by day, we have been training the mind to focus on the present moment. Although the formal sitting practice we are going to learn in this chapter is important, meditation doesn't have to be just sitting down and focusing the mind on the breath or a prayer or word. Meditation is working to be present 24/7. This is something in which warriors have been well trained. But meditation is making an effort to be present with what *is,* in *this* moment, which, a good percentage of the time—outside a war zone—does not involve a threatening element. Although any moment can be unpredictable, when we work with meditation, we can create a safe and predictable environment for ourselves.

The more we focus on what *is,* and the more we appreciate what *is,* the more time we can actually spend in the present moment. And since the present moment is *all that there really is,* the more time we spend there, the more satisfying our life can be. What about those times when the present moment isn't all that comfortable, and we would just as soon not be here? Well, it is still *all there is.* As a warrior, you have trained for war. You are prepared, so even under artillery fire or mortar attack, you are ready. The moment may be exhilarating or terrifying or both, but it is still *all there is* in that moment. When our mind is fully present, our attention completely here, then our prana is fully present, and we thus have full capacity to direct this prana toward whatever it is we wish to do. We learn that our FOB is right here, right now, all the time. If you are starting to get the hang of how yoga helps you find your own way to a healthy civilian existence, you may be wondering what this next step, meditation, is going to accomplish.

Often, when flashing back to a traumatic event and re-experiencing it, the thoughts just seem to pop up out of the subconscious with a will of their own. But you are probably starting to see, after months of practice and after your work with yoga nidra, that you *can* develop some control of the mind. The more you are able to lock your mind and body into the present moment, the more the wild and erratic thoughts of a mind shocked by trauma begin to soften and dissolve. It really is possible to change and take control of the way the brain works! By directing the mind to focus on one thing, like the breath, or the word *space,* for example, other activities in the mind—like thinking of past experiences—just don't get the juice, and they begin to settle down. In directing the mind to concentrate on whatever it is you are trying to do, you are training the brain cells—just as you would train for deployment or to run a marathon—to function efficiently, conserve energy, and follow a protocol. The neurons that are jumping around and are responsible for making all the noisy and stressful thoughts have no option but to fall in line behind the guy going at the slower pace.

More than anything, meditation is the process of sitting quietly, going deeply within, and just *observing* the activity of the mind, because as we try to focus on our breath, a mantra or word, or a prayer, thoughts will interrupt—frequently! Those noisy neurons will jump up and start swinging around, like a monkey from one tree to another. It is important to make friends with this process and not get frustrated by it, not judge the thoughts as "good" or "bad," not try to suppress them, not engage with them, not have a conversation with ourselves about how bad we are at meditation, not do anything really but observe whatever happens to come up from the depths of the mind. This is how meditation continues to help us accomplish our return to a healthy, civilian existence.

HOW MEDITATION HELPS

Practicing meditation will help you to learn that things come and go, and that is the way life is. Life is about change, endless change. When we sit for meditation every day, for just ten to fifteen minutes, we begin to see that endless change isn't such a bad thing. We sit and watch the endless panorama of experience that parades before us. And we begin to realize that everything is impermanent. The only immutable constant is the underlying Source of all things, of which we are all a part. Once we can have that experience, of really *knowing* that we are not separate and that we are all connected, then we don't feel so isolated or lonely. And that *experience* is the *experience* of yoga itself.

Meditation has a physiological component, a blueprint, and is not merely some intangible experience of "space that cannot be measured." There are some very real measurable changes that occur during meditation that have now been documented in hundreds and hundreds of studies. Like the practice of asana, and as we have experienced with pranayama and yoga nidra, meditation is a continuation of learning to access and activate the relaxation response. The pulse actually does slow down, the respiration slows, the muscles relax, the fight-or-flight response is quieted, the mind is less busy, and thoughts diminish. So the relaxation, quieting, and calming or energizing effect you feel is real.

How deeply you are able to relax and how quiet your mind becomes depend on how deep your meditation takes you. There are many stages of meditation, which can be light and shallow or heavy and deep, much like the experiences in yoga nidra. You can have the sensation of dropping way down to a very still place, or you might feel as if you are just bobbing below the surface of the threshold between sleeping and waking. Meditation, like yoga nidra, is an effortless place. Ironically, you cannot *try* to meditate. The minute you *try*, the experience disappears. It is comical. You have a moment of feeling like you are getting it! You get excited. What happens? Poof! It evaporates instantly. You just have to allow the experience of meditation to float down and descend upon you. The more you can relax and melt and let go, the more ethereal the experience becomes, and the closer you move to meditation itself.

When we are working with a meditation technique, like any of those that follow, we are in a completely *open system*. No breath control. No locks. Just open breathing-with-awareness and connecting to the world. This is exactly the opposite of the *closed systems* we put in place in our asana and pranayama practices. Instead of closing down our energetic field for purposes of purification, in meditation we think of ourselves as an open field of energy in dynamic exchange with the universe around us, which in reality is what we truly are. Universal energy flows in and out, and we join with that. We lose the sense of the individual "I" and work toward wholeness with all beings everywhere.

The three meditation techniques that follow help quiet our mind, heal our body, and conserve and focus our energy so we don't spend so much time trying to manipulate things to the way we wish they would be. We slowly, slowly learn that *this is it!* As my buddy Jon Kabat-Zinn, creator of the Stress Reduction Clinic and the Center for Mindfulness in Medicine at the University of Massachusetts, says, "There are no better moments; there are only moments." The only place we can possibly ever really be is here and now, whether we are happy or depressed, mowing the lawn or shoveling snow, in a war zone or at home. Whether we are comfortable or uncomfortable with what is going on might be important to us, but really is irrelevant in the big picture. Life is life. It is the way it is. Mindfulness is to be here in each moment, with whatever is going on, and as much of the time as possible, because this is where, and only where, life is truly lived.

This can be difficult to accept if you have just returned from combat or a war zone. There may be health issues, or uncertainty around your family situation or your work duties, but nothing can compare with the unpredictability of the environment you just left. Things seem pretty tame. It can feel boring, worthless, mundane. *Is this really the way people who aren't in the military live?* you might think. "Home" may not seem the same. It isn't—and you aren't—the same. But take comfort in the fact that *nothing* else is the same either. Nothing stays the same—ever.

All these thoughts are okay. You can sit back in a secure and grounded body as if you were in a comfortable hammock or easy chair, and just watch. Watch what comes up. What are you thinking about? See if you can just watch these thoughts without becoming glued to them. Imagine they are like clouds floating by in the sky. They will pass by.

Meditation quiets the mind and reveals the depth of human potential that resides in the heart of the soul. These techniques will come to be faithful friends, as they have been for thousands of years to many, many people just like you. Although there are countless books and opinions about the different kinds of meditation and their respective benefits and objectives, I feel strongly that the practice of meditation is more important than the meditation technique you eventually select to work with. There are many, many authentic meditation techniques—some focused on stress reduction and some pointed at realizing the Self. Any one of them can be a suitable vehicle to ferry you across to the land of quiet mind. It is important to pick a meditation technique that you like and that resonates with your spirit, and then stick with it. It's okay to spend some time trying out different practices, but jumping from technique to technique will not take you to the depth of possibility that the practice of meditation is designed to create. Eventually you want to settle on one.

PREPARATION FOR MEDITATION

Just as with asana practice, the way in which we prepare ourselves and our space for meditation is important. Here are some things to keep in mind.

Environment

To prepare for any of the meditation techniques that follow, it is important to select an environment with the least potential for distraction, and one that feels safe and relatively predictable. You want to select a space that supports your intention to be quiet, peaceful, and tuned in to your True Self. This might mean that before you begin, you close the door to your room or turn off the phone. You might want to make a place for photos or flowers or candles, or your favorite spiritual books, or whatever is sacred and meaningful to you. I like pinecones and stones and acorns and feathers I find on hikes. They help me to feel connected to nature.

Temperature

It is also important to be warm and comfortable. But you don't want to fall asleep, so this doesn't mean you should curl up on the couch under a blanket. To stay warm, you might place a blanket or jacket around your shoulders.

Your Seat

You may sit on a cushion on the floor or on a straight-backed chair, but either way, make sure that the seat is flat and not tilting forward or backward or to one side or another. If you are sitting in a chair, make sure that your feet are flat on the floor. If you are sitting on the floor, sit with your legs crossed comfortably in front of you in easy posture or any other sitting posture that is comfortable. It is best to have your hips slightly higher than your knees. This might require placing an additional pillow under your buttocks to make yourself more comfortable. Sit quietly with the spine erect. If you are in a chair, do not lean back. If you are not able to sit due to injury or pain, then lie down, flat on your back on a warm floor, perhaps on a mat or rug. You may put a very small pillow under your head. Your chin should be level with your forehead.

Posture

Sit in a posture that helps you present a noble image of yourself to yourself. Allow the spine to lengthen, with the chest lifted and the back held straight. This keeps the heart center open and receptive, and the position of the spine allows for the unimpeded movement of energy. In whatever posture you take, it is important to maintain alertness, but at the same time to be relaxed. If you are in pain, it will not be as easy to keep your attention on the object of your meditation practice. Think about your asana practice for a minute. You look to find a place of poise between hard and soft, strength and flexibility, between maintaining stability and surrendering to flow. In yoga terminology that is called balancing between *sthira* and *sukha*, or between "directed steadiness" and "ease or comfort." These are the two elements of all our yoga practices that we are looking to balance. In asana, for example, sometimes we push too hard and fall on our faces. Sometimes we don't push hard enough, and we fall asleep. Just as in your asana practice the perfect balance between the two is found through practice and paying attention, so in meditation, it is important to find that balance between tension and ease.

Close your eyes. Notice any physical discomfort zones that might be taking your attention. Try to adjust them or work them out. Then reset yourself and get comfortable again. Rest your hands palms down on your knees or one hand in the other, palms facing up in your lap, with the thumbs just touching. Relax your jaw so your mouth is almost open, with the tongue relaxed and resting just behind the back of the upper teeth. Notice any restlessness. Take a few minutes to settle in.

Meditation Practice 1 Conscious Breathing

(10 minutes)

This is a simple and powerful technique that can be used by almost anyone at any time to relax, recharge, or reconnect with the present moment. *Conscious breathing* is the process of sitting comfortably, allowing the attention to rest on the breath, like a bird rests on the branch of a tree. The technique directs our attention to present time by turning our focus to our breath. Conscious breathing is an easy way to get grounded and centered. It affords us the opportunity to slow down and get in touch with just exactly what *is,* whatever that might be at the moment. It helps us to notice just exactly what we are doing with our prana, or life force.

As we sit, we start to realize again and again, as we have begun to do with our previous practices, that we can watch our thoughts, as something apart from our *self,* as we might watch a movie. We begin to notice the exact moment when we are distracted from the object of our concentration, which in this case is the breath. We might still be breathing, but once we become distracted and start thinking about something, we have forgotten about our breath, and are no longer *consciously breathing.* In meditation, we are conscious of our breathing but, unlike pranayama, we are not controlling it. The more we practice this conscious watching, the more we realize how much of the time we are *not here mentally!* In this practice, we learn to recognize and make friends with this incessant chatter of the mind that we call *thought.* We allow ourselves to simply watch the mental festivities, without judging or engaging with them, and then return our attention to our breath. When we see a thought bubble up from the depths and pop up on the screen of our mind, we learn to recognize the thought as just thought. Not good or bad thought, but just thought. We discover that we can pull our attention back from the past or the future and delightfully return to our breath and the present moment.

This is an uncomplicated practice that prepares us for more advanced meditation techniques. However, it is *not only* a practice for beginners. Even those who have practiced meditation for thirty or forty years can benefit from this technique, simply because this kind of work is so important and so easy.

The following preliminary instructions are given as a way to help you ease into each of the three meditation techniques given in this chapter. The preparation is similar to the way you prepare for your pranayama practice. So familiarize yourself with the general procedure of settling in and getting quiet. I won't take the time to repeat these instructions in detail for each of the practices that follow. Feel free to add to the process any personal prayer or ritual that may help you come to rest and commit to your meditation practice. Please remember that in meditation you are working with an *open system*. There is no control of the breath, no locks, no external gazing point. The eyes are closed, there is only effortless effort, and our gaze now is internal—we are looking in!

Preliminary Practice: Settling In

Come to a comfortable seated position. Close your eyes. Take a few deep breaths. Notice any physical discomfort that might be taking your attention. Make any necessary adjustments to your seat or posture so you can be comfortable. Settle in.

Notice the surrounding environment. Imagine a radar beam, shining out from your center, circling around 360 degrees, scanning the external environment. What is going on today? Take notice. Is there sound? Traffic? Wind? Neighbors? Listen objectively. Again, try not to judge the sounds as good sounds or bad sounds. Just listen. Let them be. Accept them as part of what *is* for this moment. Notice the smell of the room, the feel of the air on your skin. Sit with this.

Now turn the radar beam to point in, and scan the internal environment. Pull your attention inward and observe what is going on there. Are you bored? Restless? Depressed? Excited? Irritated? Rerunning an event from earlier in the day? Who or what is taking your attention? Don't try to suppress or judge your thoughts. Let them bubble up from the floor of the unconscious mind. Watch your thoughts as though they were leaves floating by on the surface of a river. As you sit on the banks of the river, watch them as they pass by, in and out of view.

Conscious Breathing

Now gently shift your attention to your natural breath. Just like that, begin to rest the attention on the breath. Although it is impossible to look at anything without changing it, now that you are noticing your breath, the tendency is to take control of it. Instead, be aware of that, and change it as little as possible. Just watch. Tune into the natural movement of your breath, the rising and falling of the belly. (Remember, you are just watching your natural breath now, not using ujjayi breathing or any other pranayama technique.) Feel the breath as it moves in and out of the body, and feel the sensations in your body that accompany the breath. Let your attention descend on the breath like leaves fluttering to the ground in autumn, gently falling and covering the breath.

When you become distracted by a sound, or a sensation, or a thought, gently bring yourself back to your breath. You cannot force the attention on to the breath. You must simply allow it to rest there, like the air is simply there, touching you. Let your attention be like the air—gentle and effortless, no struggle. Just relax, as if you were falling toward sleep, but you do not fall asleep. The mind is alert and happy to rest on the breath.

Where is your attention now? If you notice that a thought has distracted you, just bring your attention back to your breath. Just like that. Don't get mad at your mind. Just acknowledge the thought. And again, bring the attention to touch the breath. Be patient and kind with yourself. Over time, you will experience difficult days and more easy ones— stay with it. You will slowly learn how to calm and center yourself using the breath. Let the tension dissolve from the body. Let any tightness give way to buoyancy. Let yourself melt into relaxation and conscious breathing, but keep your posture erect and upright. Every time the mind drifts off and you lose contact with the breath, patiently bring your attention back to the movement of the breath in your body. Stay with this practice for ten minutes.

Returning to Waking Consciousness

Slowly now, begin your return journey to waking consciousness, becoming aware of the sounds around you, the smell in the room, a taste, perhaps, in your mouth. Begin—slowly— to move, twisting lightly first to the right and then to the left. Keep your eyes closed and, if you like, rub your hands together for a few seconds, and then rest your closed eyes in the palms of your hands. Gently, open your eyes, halfway at first. Let your hands fall slowly away, allowing the outside world to gradually return, then fully take in the light and the space around you. At a leisurely pace, return to the world you left. Smile. Say thank you. Be grateful for this time and for all that you have. Carry this awareness with you for the rest of the day.

When to Practice

This is an excellent practice to do first thing in the morning or just before bed. It can be done before or after prayer, or when you need to anchor down and get centered and grounded. Conscious breathing can actually be used anywhere, any time, to create a sense of control and put you in touch with your Self. It is very similar to the practice that follows. You can try both of them and pick the one that works best for you. However, if you are working regularly with a pranayama technique and it is helping you—whether to sleep, relax, de-stress, calm your emotions, or whatever—then stick with that. All yoga students struggle with the following question: "How will I juggle asana practice, pranayama, and meditation, and get them all in—along with my work, my family obligations, my time for myself, my running or swimming or biking or working out in the gym . . . ." Whoa! One breath at a time. Do what you can. It's all good. When there is time for a little extra, you can add in the meditations early in the morning or before bedtime.

Meditation Practice 2
Japa Yoga—the Repetition of a Word or Prayer

(12–15 minutes)

This is a simple technique that has been used by yoga practitioners for thousands of years. It is also a continuation of the conscious breathing technique, in that it adds a word or a prayer or phrase to the focus on the breath, and is very similar to the technique that Herbert Benson teaches in his book, *The Relaxation Revolution*. The use of a word or prayer or mantra for meditation is referred to in yoga as the practice of *japa*, which means "recitation" and refers to the mental repetition of the word or mantra as a point for focus. This should then lead naturally to the contemplation of the inner significance of the prayer or word.

Progressive Relaxation

Come to your comfortable sitting position. Settle in. Relax all the muscles in your body. Start with your feet, and then taking a minute or so, mentally move up through the body, from the feet, to the calves, the thighs, the pelvis, and on up, consciously focusing on and relaxing each portion of your body. When you get to your shoulders and neck, continue up and relax the face, the scalp, and the jaw.

Natural Breath

Now focus your attention on your natural breath. Do not try to control or change your breath. Just watch it rise and fall, in and out for a few moments. Take time to notice a few things about your natural breath. Where do you feel it? High or low in your body? Is it deep or shallow? Is it fast or slow? Warm or cool? Dry or humid? Just notice and make a note to yourself. There is no good or better pattern. Tomorrow it will change.

Select a Phrase, Word, or Prayer

Next, pick a word or phrase or your favorite prayer or mantra or even an image, such as the face of Jesus or Buddha. The word can be secular, such as *space* or *peace* or *light* or *joyful;* or it can be spiritual, such as *God is One* or *Hail Mary, full of Grace* or *One Spirit* or *Om mani padme hum* (the Tibetan mantra meaning roughly "the jewel in the heart of the lotus"). Take five seconds, and select the first thing that comes to you that is in some way spiritually uplifting for you. Don't make an enormous Hollywood production out of selecting your word or prayer. Something will pop into your mind—use that unless it is really not appropriate. Tomorrow you can find something else, but for now, just use whatever it is that comes to you.

Japa Practice

Begin now to direct your attention to your exhalation. Then every time you exhale, mentally repeat your word or phrase. Let yourself feel as if you are placing the word (or prayer or image) on the exhalation, connecting the word to the breath. If you are using a single word, draw it out over the length of the exhalation. If you are using a short prayer, then it might spill over into the inhalation.

Imagine, if you like, that you are pouring or loading your word onto your exhale. Allow your exhalation to carry the word down through the center of yourself, like an elevator or a breaking wave. For me, it often happens that my word becomes like a waterfall, actually *becomes* a waterfall, flowing over a cliff and falling down into a clear blue stream below. The visual image of the water that I see in my mind just carries the word over the edge into my exhalation.

When your mind wanders off and you are distracted, which will happen over and over again, simply notice, and take a mental attitude of shrugging your shoulders and saying silently to yourself, "Thinking" or "Oh, well," and then bring your attention back to your word, and again, continue to repeat the word and lay it over your exhalation.

It is important to be relaxed about your distractions. You will get distracted. Everyone gets distracted. It's not a big deal, and it isn't good or bad—it's just a distraction. The essential thing is to notice that you have been distracted and to bring your attention back. Just like that. No agita! Set a timer and sit like this for ten or twelve minutes.

Returning with a Visualization

When your chime goes off, indicating that your meditation period is ending, take a couple minutes to visualize a situation or condition or environment that you would like to bring about for yourself. Perhaps it is to be healthy or healed from a current injury, or to move to a home in the countryside, or to have a joyful family environment. Whatever it is, imagine that it is already happening. Create a statement, as you did for setting your intention, your sankalpa, in yoga nidra. It should be in the first-person, present tense, like "With awareness, I am creating healthy habits," or "My mind and body flow in perfect harmony," or "I use my energy to heal and transform." Visualize yourself in that environment. Take time to see where you are. Are you alone or is someone there with you? Are you with friends? Are you outside? Inside? Imagine the way you will actually *feel* when this situation becomes manifest. Take your time. Try and get in touch with the feeling you are having, knowing that this condition or situation is actually already happening and is *here* and *now*.

Close this image by saying thank you and feeling grateful for something that you do have. Slowly return to full waking consciousness. Take your time to reenter the space around you. Do this every day for the next month. Then take note of what effect it has.

Meditation Practice 3 Walking Meditation

(20–30 minutes)

I learned this walking meditation technique from Thich Nhat Hanh, a Vietnamese Buddhist monk, and the following instructions are drawn from his book *Walking Meditation*. I have found this practice to be really helpful when I feel like I am getting close to overload or caught up in a huge wave that's tumbling forward, rolling me over and over, out of control. For the moment, I feel helpless and am not able to take charge of the turmoil I feel building. It's not a great feeling.

At times like this, when you feel like you are on the edge of losing it, it can be hard to just sit and try to meditate. This is a way to take action, but slow down at the same time.

What is Walking Meditation?

Walking meditation is the practice of simply walking—slowly and mindfully. The purpose is to completely enjoy the experience of walking. It's walking just to walk, rather than walking to get somewhere, which is how we generally walk. We take the time to enjoy each step, to appreciate the support that our earth gives us each time we take a step. We mindfully set down each foot, then pick it up and set down the other foot as we breathe and relax and appreciate the moment. We are not trying to arrive anywhere, and our destination is simply the here and now.

Thich Nhat Hanh described it well in his book.

> In the midst of our chaotic world, we tend to lose touch with the peace and joy that are available in each moment: the sunshine, the birds' singing, the autumn leaves, a baby's smile. The practice of walking meditation brings us back to being fully present and alive with every step, filling each moment with peace and joy.

He goes on to explain that walking meditation helps us to slow down and relax, drawing our attention off our worries and anxieties about the past or the future and bringing our attention to the present moment. Often we don't want to be in the present moment because it is uncomfortable or unpleasant or worse. We tend to think that there is nothing here for us now except pain and suffering. But if we just take a step and a breath, and ask the earth and the wind and the trees to help us in taking this one step in a gentle moment, free of struggle, perhaps then we can take another step, and another.

Walking meditation can be done inside or outside. If you are walking inside you can take off your shoes, if you like. And even if you are walking outside, on the grass or in the woods or on the beach, it's great if you can take off your shoes. Of course, it depends on where you are walking and on the time of year. But if you are barefoot, you can feel the floor or the ground and connect directly with the earth. No matter where you live, you can almost always find a small fragment of nature to help you to get through your struggle. You are reminded that the air and the birds and the trees and forests and rivers are always there for you. Every time you take a slow, mindful step, it reminds you that Mother Earth is here for you, supporting you in this moment.

The longer you practice this mindful, slow walking, the more you will be able to relax and open your heart and find the joyfulness in each moment. This might sound a little silly at first, and if you are going through a troublesome time, the whole idea of using walking to help you "get through" and find a bit of peace might seem absurd. But if you will simply take the first step, and then another, and another, and actually do this step by step—not in a hurry to find relief, not as something to rush through, but just to walk, you will find that transformation happens.

Walking Meditation Practice

Find a starting point. Set a realistic goal. Perhaps you will only take ten steps today or walk for ten minutes. As you put time aside for this practice, you will find that you miss it when you don't do it and will look forward to returning to the peacefulness of walking meditation.

The pace is very slow and deliberate. Each foot is placed mindfully down, as you follow the roll of the foot as it touches down and then pushes off. It is easier to do when you are by yourself or with friends out in nature than on a busy sidewalk in New York City. But in either case, it is possible to walk mindfully. You can hold your hands together behind your back or fold them together in front of you as you walk. Do what is comfortable and easy. To help coordinate your breathing with your walking, you can practice either by counting your breath or by using words. Breathe in, step, breathe out, step. Or perhaps you will breathe in for two steps and out for two steps. Follow the natural rhythm of your breath. By coordinating your breath with your steps, you anchor your attention in the present moment. You don't want to speed up the breath so you can walk faster or make it a military-type march. It is gentle and flowing. If you can synchronize your breath with your steps, then do that, but if not, let it all go and relax. Just return your attention to your desire to be relaxed and calm and joyful.

If you want to coordinate words to your breathing pattern, you can say silently, as Thich Nhat Hanh suggests, "I touch the earth gently, I touch the earth gently," or "The sun, the sky, the trees. The sun, the sky, the trees," as you walk. Or say anything you like that is soothing and beautiful to you. Say hello to the things you see. Smile at the blue sky. Every path can be a walking meditation path, along a road, in the woods, through a village, or through a bustling city. When you do walking meditation in a busy city, you can walk the same way that you do when you are out in nature. You may not see as many birds or trees, but you can still walk peacefully amid the noise and turbulence. Since you are in a public place and you don't want to attract attention from people who are wondering what in the world you are doing, you might want to walk a little bit faster than your "out in nature" walking.

When you first begin to walk this slowly, you may feel a little off balance. This is pretty normal as you are not used to this slow pace. Gradually, it will become easier. As you step, take time to feel the earth under your feet. Feel grounded. This will help you to find balance.

Breathing in, "Good morning birds." Breathing out, "Thank you for your songs." Or, breathing in, "Good morning bicycles." Breathing out, "Thank you for sharing the road." Allow your whole body to relax into every step and feel the rhythm of your breath harmonize with the rhythm of the earth.

Maybe you stop along the way and simply breathe or take time to look more carefully at some one thing—a tree or a spider who is busy spinning her web or a sparkling stream. You will notice things you never noticed before and find yourself wrapped up in a world that often escapes us as we hurry from place to place. We realize that it is all there for us to enjoy. As you continue to breathe consciously, you feel peaceful and move on, one mindful step at a time.

As Thich Nhat Hanh says:

> Doing walking meditation in this way helps us mend our hearts. Life has not been easy for many of us, and oftentimes our hearts have been torn and broken. But as we learn to walk mindfully, coming home to the Earth with each step, we mend our broken hearts. Every step you take in this spirit becomes a healing stitch that mends the places in you that are wounded.

ESTABLISHING A DAILY MEDITATION PRACTICE

Awareness of the breath is the fundamental technique of these three practices and of most meditation practices in general. Which technique you use—whether conscious breathing, or japa practice with conscious breathing, or walking meditation, or even any other mindfulness meditation practice—doesn't really matter so much. What matters is your commitment to sit, or if you choose walking meditation, your commitment to walk. There are a few things you can do to help you establish a daily meditation practice.

- Plan to meditate at the same time every day. As with pranayama, it can be best to sit right after you get up in the morning, or after a shower, or a cup of tea or coffee. The earlier it is, the less active your mind will be, and the easier it will be to settle down. If you can't get to it in the morning, then get to it whenever you can. But make an effort to be consistent in your time. This may seem unimportant and/or difficult at first, but it can help make your practice more regular.

- Find a quiet place where you can feel safe and comfortable. Wherever it is, pick a place where you can be relatively undisturbed.

- Create a meditation space, perhaps with a photo of an inspiring image or person, or personal objects that are special or sacred to you. Or bring a book from which you can read a short inspiring passage before you start.

- Keep it simple. You are not necessarily trying to induce a particular state of mind but just trying to bring clarity to whatever it is you are experiencing in the moment.

Try out each technique and see what works for you. One or another may come to be more comfortable and appropriate, or more effective, than the others, in which case you should focus, for your formal practice, on that particular technique. Intermittently you might even want to search around for a guided meditation tape for a specific effect or to retrain your brain, so to speak, or to get reprogrammed, and make sure you are on the right track. Every time you study these methods, whether those given here or any authentic meditation techniques, you will gain a deeper understanding of the practice.

Over the past few months, this meditation has helped me realize how closely connected my physical and mental pain are. I told my wife that I feel like I'm untangling a big knot. I didn't know which strand was which when it was all knotted together, but as I do the meditation, I feel myself unwinding. As I undo the knot, I see what was mental and what was physical and how letting go of each helps the other.

VIETNAM VETERAN

CHAPTER 10

SEEKING HIGHER SELF

THE JOURNEY WITHIN

Yoga is simple. It only takes a little attention, a little practice every day, and soon we realize we have developed a regular practice. We meditate for ten or fifteen minutes every morning; we do a regular asana practice. We use the breathing exercises or a yoga nidra recording to relax and calm the mind. Slowly, we start to notice that we are sleeping a little better, or that we are a little more patient, a little calmer, a little more content, a little less grumpy or reactive or jumpy. We slowly realize that *practice* in the yogic sense of the word simply means "making an effort to keep the mind steady," to be *here*, wherever *here* might be. It dawns on us that we can *practice* all the time, 24/7, that it doesn't matter what we are doing, and that when we are making an effort to be present, no matter what is going on, it limits the drama, the saga, the memories, the story our mind wants to press upon us.

There is no room in our mind to reexperience past events or worry about the future if we just get our attention into present time, hold it there, and find something in that present time that we can be grateful for, or attend to, or smile about. And when we can't find something to smile about, we can breathe! And soon, *this too will pass,* whatever *this* might have been, and we can smile again. We can *learn* to turn on the relaxation response instead of the fight-or-flight response. We can learn to control our mind!

Once we have worked through the early stage of yoga, which is basically the physical practice of asana, a change begins to happen. If we have made even the smallest effort to pay attention, some tiny seed sprouts imperceptibly and begins to grow. With continued practice, a natural evolution occurs from gross to subtle, from the physical to the spiritual, from lesser awareness to greater awareness. Once this happens, we begin to *consciously* change. Change is happening all the time, every nanosecond, but this change is being consciously directed by *us.* It can take from six months to six lifetimes, but at some point, with regular practice—and there is absolutely no doubt about this—a process we call *waking up* starts to unfold.

Since yoga is about paying attention and getting our attention into present time, there may be an instant when the mind becomes still. In that moment of stillness, there is a glimpse of a deeper reality, a peek at something beyond thought, when the attention comes to rest in the now—a moment of recognition that we are organically connected to wholeness, a moment that goes beyond deliberations and worries over the past and future, a real glimpse of pure awareness that transcends time and space. If the experience is profound enough, there will be an actual spiritual experience of the true yoga itself, an experience of what is often called the *True Self,* or the revelation of nonduality, or the idea that there is nothing other than *One.* Our fears of nonbeing, of dying, of separateness and loneliness become less profound as we start to sense our oneness and connectedness to the whole shebang, to our fellow humans, to all beings everywhere, even to what we might refer to as God. The light dawns; that's it! We come to realize through our practice that the yoga methodology is one path (although not the only path) that offers a map that can take us to the destination and reveal to us how we truly are connected to one another.

The idea of an underlying oneness, or a connectedness, is not new. We can look back into the history of all ancient cultures and indigenous peoples and find a tradition of nonduality. Even science these days is looking behind the diversity of all the forms in our universe and seeking a unity to it all. Fundamental to quantum theory in the field of physics, for example, and one of the most significant parallels between the world of science and the ancient yoga teachings, is this idea of nonlocality, or *connectedness*. Quantum interconnectedness is the idea that two quanta (very tiny particles) of energy, which are not in proximity (not touching or nearly touching), are still connected! An experiment that proved this and has been repeated often demonstrates that two quanta of light called *photons,* shot off from a single source and traveling at the speed of light in opposite directions, can maintain their connection to one another. In this experiment, any effect placed on one photon as it rockets away from the other registers instantaneously with the other. What happens to one happens to the other. Pretty amazing! But not so amazing to the ancient yogis who have known this all along.

And exactly how did the yogis and *rishis* (spiritual adepts) come to know this thousands of years ago, we may wonder? Well, without the World Wide Web and Google search, we can imagine that they came to this awareness through a profound inner revelation. Many people have a deep knowing of the connectedness that transcends the physical world. Surely many military service people during a combat mission have had indescribable experiences of unity with all that is—as well as moments of truly knowing God.

Once we truly realize this connection, even for an instant, we begin to care about the world around us and about the people in it because we realize that there really is only one of us here. This realization is the endgame of yoga. As it says in the Bible a "peace that surpasses all understanding" (Philippians 4:7) begins to descend upon us. By "surpassing" understanding, the Christian scriptures are telling us that the experience goes beyond the understanding, or the conceptualization of the *idea* of peace. Instead it is a *feeling* of peace inside our heart, not just a thought in our mind.

Peace isn't something we hope happens out there somewhere in the world. Peace begins with us, right here, right now. Our developing yoga practice helps us to find the ability and skills to remain clear and calm in the midst of life's challenges and stresses. We can then work effectively to transform internal discord and violence into cooperation and peace, not only within ourselves, but within our family and community as well. Yoga helps us to free ourselves from the habit of constant worry and stressful thinking, which leads to disappointment, unhappiness, fear, and suffering as a way of life. It is an empowering practice that puts much of our health and well-being into our own hands.

And it can help us to break from the uniquely human pattern of thinking that who we are in any moment is whatever we happen to be thinking about. Instead, we learn that at every moment we have a choice: we can be swept along by the winds of change and by our thought processes or we can anchor down to our True Self. Developing our practices is certainly one way that can help us to stay connected to the True Self that exists beyond thought. But walking through woods where we feel safe or along the seashore, being out in nature, listening to beautiful music, or creating or appreciating magnificent art, these can also be experiences that give us the feeling of connectedness with Being or One Spirit.

There is no way to really describe what we mean by *being*. It is a state of oneness, of what Eckhart Tolle, in his book *The Power of Now,* calls "aware presence." It is a sense of recognition of who we truly are from deep within ourselves. Our Being is the knower behind the thinker, our innermost indestructible essence. Once we begin to realize, through our yoga and meditation practice, that our thoughts are not who we are, but instead are actually something that we can sit back and watch, and choose to change if we wish, then we start to have a clue about *who* that knower behind the thinker might be. We see that as we quiet our mind, it is our body, rather than the mind, that can serve as a dependable point of access to our innermost Being. By disengaging from thoughts, observing our breathing, and connecting with deeper energetic sensations in our body, we can see ourselves and the present moment as they truly are, free from the mind's interpretations. Our Being is divine. This is the greatest teaching of yoga.

A key to being at peace is to accept what is. The minute we offer resistance to the present moment, we are out of touch; and anytime we try to argue with reality, we are going to lose! Not resisting, though, doesn't mean (as I have mentioned a few times) sitting back and accepting anything that comes down the pike. It also does not mean not doing anything, or not taking action. It means accepting this moment, as it is, whether we like it or not, as opposed to *reacting* to it. If we are stuck in the mud, the first thing we need to do is acknowledge that we are stuck in the mud. If we thrash and flail around, we get stuck even deeper. But if we first accept the fact that we are stuck in the mud, we can begin our civilian land nav and plot our next move. The next moment, things can change. Things will change. We can take action to direct the course of the next moment.

In yoga, the ability to respond to a situation mindfully and correctly is referred to as *right action*. It has nothing to do with the speed of response. Right action can be immediate, and often is, or it can require time and deliberation. Our ability to develop appropriate right action comes through the skillful means we cultivate through our right practice. As we work to still the mind, all the clouds disappear. Clear sky appears, and we see truly; the right action that needs to be taken is evident.

So to all of you reading this book—warriors all, veterans and military service men and women who have gone through war and combat—the inspiring and joyful moments and the friendships you gained, as well as the difficulties, the bad memories, and the traumas you experienced, have all contributed to who you are in this moment. As you grow older, it becomes easier to think of your most painful moments as opportunities for your growth, and you can begin to see how they can help you to understand life in all its complexities and challenges. You are warriors. You have accomplished much—many things that others will never do or understand. I hope this system of yoga will help you to direct your strength and courage inward in the battle to conquer the inner enemies, guide you on the path to the peace of mind we all seek, and be of assistance as you find your own way to a healthy, happy, and purposeful life living as a warrior in a noncombat zone—in other words, living at *home* once again. Breathe in, breathe out. That's all.

WHAT DO THOSE SANSKRIT WORDS MEAN?

asana The physical yoga postures, or poses, intended to
create strength, flexibility, and balance; traditionally
regarded as the gateway to and preparation for
meditation; the third of the eight limbs of yoga.

astanga Eight-limbed yoga (*ashto* means "eight" and
anga means "limb"); the path of yoga outlined in
the ancient text, *The Yoga Sutra,* which lays out how
a person can achieve inner peace and knowledge
through yoga in eight steps. The eight limbs are **yama**
(restraint), **niyama** (observance), **asana** (posture),
pranayama (breath work), **pratyahara** (withdrawal
of the senses), **dharana** (concentration), **dhyana**
(meditation), and **samadhi** (self-realization).

bandha An energetic lock that guides the flow of
energy in yoga practice; the two focused on in this
book are **mula bandha** and **uddiyana bandha.**

dharana Concentration; the effort to hold the
mind's attention on a single thought or a
spot; the sixth of the eight limbs of yoga.

dhyana Meditation; contemplation; the continuous flow of awareness between the meditator and the object of meditation as the mind remains focused and expanded into quietness; the seventh of the eight limbs of yoga.

japa Repetition; repeating a sacred prayer or phrase over and over.

mantra A sacred sound or prayer to focus on to still the mind in meditation.

mula bandha The energetic root lock engaged during yoga practice; a process that initially requires consciously "locking" or tightening and physically lifting up the floor of the pelvis and that eventually is accomplished through energetic awareness.

niyama Observance; five principles to guide our personal conduct: saucha (purity, cleanliness), santosa (contentment), **tapas** (the burning of toxins through austerities involving self-discipline and the desire to purify the body, senses, and mind), svadhyaya (self-study, study of both the scriptures and one's own body, mind, intellect, and ego), and Ishvara pranidhana (devotion, surrender to the God of your understanding or to pure awareness); the second of the eight limbs of yoga.

om Referred to in yoga as *pranava,* or the "unstruck" sound; a vibration or sound representing absolute divine consciousness or pure awareness; can be used as a *bija* (seed) mantra.

Patanjali The sage who wrote *The Yoga Sutra*, the two thousand-plus-year-old text delineating classical yoga and outlining the eight limbs.

prana Energy; life force; the energy that permeates all forms of consciousness, from the individual to all living beings and life forms, as well as all things everywhere, from stones to planets to stars and beyond.

pranayama Control of the breath; expansion (*ayama*) of the inner life force energy (**prana**) through the use of conscious breathing; the fourth of the eight limbs of yoga; consists of three parts: inhalation, exhalation, and the pauses between the two.

pratyahara Withdrawal of the senses as the mind turns inward from physical poses and breath work; the fifth of the eight limbs of yoga.

Raja Yoga The yoga of psycho/physical exercise; one of four types of yoga; also referred to as Classical yoga and astanga yoga; translates literally as "royal yoga." See **astanga.**

rajasic Active; when used in reference to the yoga postures, it refers to an active yoga practice, as opposed to a more quiet or restorative practice.

samadhi A state of total absorption experienced through Self-Realization and the experience of "yoga" itself; the final of the eight limbs of yoga. The meditation and the meditator become one, and awareness of an individual self is lost, resulting in freedom from matter and thought.

samskara A deeply stored impression (good and bad) or trauma from last week, last year, our childhood, or previous lifetime that can be released (or burned) through the practice of yoga; literally translates as "imprint"; we create samskaras every moment, and they determine the path our journey takes.

sankalpa A positive statement directed at reaching a whole life pattern, stated positively and in the present tense, for example, "I am healing and regaining health for the benefit of all beings everywhere."

sthira Steadiness; one of two qualities in yoga that should be present in all aspects of practice, from **asana** through meditation. The other is **sukha,** or ease.

sukha Ease; one of two qualities that should be present in all aspects of yoga practice, from **asana** through meditation. The other is **sthira,** or steadiness.

tapas The burning of toxins through austerities involving self-discipline and the desire to purify the body, senses, and mind; one of the **niyamas,** or observances, to guide our personal conduct.

uddiyana bandha "The fly-up lock"; the physical pulling in and up through the core muscles of the abdomen a few inches below the navel, and eventually accomplished through energetic awareness.

ujjayi Means "expand into victory;" a powerful closed-mouth breathing technique for use while practicing yoga postures or as a stand-alone **pranayama** practice to steady the mind and heat the body.

vritti A fluctuation, wave, or a thought or the "noise" of the mind, stilled through the practice of yoga.

yama Restraint; the first of the eight limbs of yoga; five principles to guide our social interactions: ahimsa (nonviolence), satya (truthfulness), asteya (non-stealing), brahamacharya (moderation, a disciplined sexual life, sometimes translated as celibacy in the case of monks), and aparigraha (nongreediness, nonpossessiveness).

yoga nidra Yogic "sleep," or sleep with a slight trace of awareness; a deep relaxation process that gradually withdraws our awareness from the outer world and turns it inward.

Yoga Sutra, The Compiled by the sage Patanjali; an ancient collection of 196 aphorisms, or short "threads" of concise wisdom; lays out in the second chapter a practical, step-by-step set of instructions on how a person can achieve inner peace and knowledge through yoga.

ACKNOWLEDGMENTS

My deepest gratitude and appreciation to the many individuals and organizations for their selfless service, hard work, publishing expertise, and mindful eyes, all of which have contributed in truly countless ways to make the publication of this book possible:

- To all our veterans and military service men and women who are the true inspiration for this work.

- To the countless yoga service organizations and studios for their selfless service to veterans and their families.

- To my teacher Munishree Chitrabhanu, the Jain monk who guided my life of spiritual inquiry through the entire decade of the 1970s, inspired me to travel to India in 1974, and taught me meditation and the principles of *ahimsa* (reverence for life) and *anakantavada* (relativity of thinking).

- To my teacher Norman Allen, who taught me the astanga vinyasa asana system in the early 1980s and first awakened me to the eight-limbed path of classical yoga, and to his teacher, Sri K. Pattabhi Jois, with whom I studied from 1987 to 1993.

- To the Give Back Yoga Foundation (a nonprofit organization whose mission is to provide yoga teachers with the resources to develop and deliver yoga programs of all types to underserved and under-resourced areas of the world, founded in 2007 by Rob Schware, Lori Klein, and me) for funding the initial expenses of copyediting, photography, and travel expenses for the models, and for partnering with Sounds True in order to make the publication of this book possible.

- Special thanks to Rob Schware, executive director of the Give Back Yoga Foundation, who shepherded this book from start to finish. His dedication to "getting it done and out" really made the completion of the book you have in your hands possible.

- To James Fox, founder of the Prison Yoga Project and author of *Yoga: A Path to Healing and Recovery,* whose book (supported and published in part by the Give Back Foundation) gave us the initial idea for this project.

- To Suzanne Manafort and Mindful Yoga Therapy for Veterans for their work and research on the use of yoga therapy and methodology in the treatment of post-traumatic stress and for help with organizing the first photo shoot for this book.

- To the eight amazing men and women, all veterans and representing the Army, Air Force, Navy, and Marine Corps, who were the models for all the yoga postures and worked tirelessly with our photographers to bring you the fabulous images in this book. Thanks Liz, Alex, Shane, John, Mike, Melinda, Phil, and Tim.

- To our incredibly talented photographers for donating their professional services to this project: Elizabeth Watts (New York City) and her assistant Maria Ferrari for all the photos in the book and Carolyn and Brian Robbins of Robbins Point Photography in Virginia Beach for the photo of Shane and for our cover photo of Liz and Alex.

- To Ann Richardson Stevens in Virginia Beach for all her help in arranging and preparing for our cover photo shoot and for donating the use of her spacious and stunning yoga studio, Studio Bamboo, to use as the location for making the beautiful image that graces the cover of this book.

- To Lori Klein, my trusted and beloved assistant of many years and director of the teacher training programs for my school, The Hard & The Soft Yoga Institute, for her focused and creative work in helping to manage the business, for her organizational and scheduling skills, for her valuable advice in every aspect of my life, and for being a great mother to her two boys, a brilliant student, and a dear friend.

And to these many others:

- To Herbert Benson, MD, for his books, *The Relaxation Response* and *Relaxation Revolution,* and his research into the health benefits of yoga and meditation.

- To Tom Steffans, Rear Admiral, US Navy (retired) and former Navy SEAL, for his first-round reading of the manuscript and his pulling-no-punches evaluation, both of which helped to make this a better book and closer to the mark for true warriors.

- To the board members of the Give Back Yoga Foundation—Anne Richardson Stevens, Suzanne Manafort, and Stan Woodman—for their support of this project.

- To Sara Neufeld, who helped to prepare the glossary of Sanskrit terms.

- To Tami Simon and Nancy Smith of Sounds True for their leap of faith.

- To the entire team at Sounds True for their amazing patience, perseverance, and persistence in getting this book finished and out and into the spectacular end result you hold in your hands—special thanks to those talented souls listed below who I had the pleasure of working with directly and to the many folks behind the scenes that I have yet to meet!

- To Jennifer Brown, senior acquisitions editor at Sounds True, for the vote of confidence to acquire *Yoga for Warriors*.

- To Jennifer Holder, editor, who first brought forward the *Yoga for Warriors* project to Sounds True, for her exceptional skill in helping to organize the manuscript.

- To Leslie Brown, production editor, who expertly shepherded the book through the various stages of production.

- To Lisa Kerans, art director, who worked incredibly hard from Boulder to pull together the cover photo shoot on the East Coast, and then (with Rachael Murray) flew to Virginia Beach to giftedly oversee and direct the project.

- To Rachael Murray, senior book designer, who took all the pieces of the project—the text and the photos—and seamlessly wove them together to produce this glorious piece of artwork that is called *Yoga for Warriors*.

SELECTED BIBLIOGRAPHY

BOOKS

Anh-Huong, Nguyen, and Thich Nhat Hanh. *Walking Meditation.* Boulder: Sounds True, 2006.

Beck, Charlotte Joko. *Everyday Zen: Love and Work.* New York: HarperCollins Publishers, 1989.

Benson, Herbert. *Relaxation Revolution.* New York: Simon and Schuster, 2010.

Benson, Herbert, and Miriam Z. Klipper. *The Relaxation Response.* New York: HarperTorch, 2000.

Birch, Beryl Bender. *Beyond Power Yoga.* New York: Simon and Schuster, 2000.

———. *Boomer Yoga.* South Portland, ME: Sellers Publishing, 2009.

———. *Power Yoga.* New York: Simon and Schuster, 1995.

Boccio, Frank Jude. *Mindfulness Yoga: The Awakened Union of Breath, Body, and Mind.* Somerville, MA: Wisdom Publications, 1993.

Boorstein, Sylvia. *Don't Just Do Something, Sit There: A Mindfulness Retreat.* New York: HarperOne, 1996.

Chödrön, Pema. *Taking the Leap: Freeing Ourselves from Old Habits and Fears.* Boston: Shambhala Publications, 2010.

———. *When Things Fall Apart: Heart Advice for Difficult Times.* Boston: Shambhala Publications, 1997.

Dalai Lama and Victor Chan. *The Wisdom of Forgiveness: Intimate Journeys and Conversations.* New York: Riverhead, 2004.

Desikachar, T. K. V. *The Heart of Yoga: Developing a Personal Practice.* Rochester, NY: Inner Traditions International, 1999.

Emerson, David, and Elizabeth Hopper, PhD. *Overcoming Trauma through Yoga.* Berkeley: North Atlantic Books, 2011.

Goldberg, Philip. *American Veda: From Emerson and the Beatles to Yoga and Meditation—How Indian Spirituality Changed the West.* New York: Harmony Books, 2010.

Hanh, Thich Nhat. *Peace Is Every Step: The Path of Mindfulness in Everyday Life.* New York: Bantam Books, 1991.

Hoge, Charles W., MD. *Once a Warrior, Always a Warrior*. Guilford, CT: GPP Life, 2010.

Iyengar, B. K. S. *Light on Yoga*. New York: Knopf Doubleday Publishing, 1995.

———. *Yoga: The Path to Holistic Health*. London: Dorling Kindersley Publishers, 2008.

Kornfield, Jack. *After the Ecstasy, the Laundry: How the Heart Grows Wise on the Spiritual Path*. New York: Bantam Books, 2000.

———. *A Path with Heart: A Guide through the Perils and Promises of Spiritual Life*. New York: Bantam Books, 1993.

———. *The Wise Heart: A Guide to the Universal Teachings of Buddhist Psychology*. New York: Bantam Dell, 2008.

Knopp, Sheldon. *If You Meet the Buddha on the Road, Kill Him!* New York: Bantam Books, 1972.

Maehle, Gregor. *Ashtanga Yoga: Practice and Philosophy*. Novata, CA: New World Library, 2007.

Mingyur Rinpoche, Yongey. *The Joy of Living*. New York: Three Rivers Press, 2007.

Mortenson, Greg, and David Olive Relin. *Three Cups of Tea: One Man's Mission to Promote Peace . . . One School at a Time*. New York: Penguin Books, 2006.

Perlmutter, David, MD, FACN, and Alberto Villoldo, PhD. *Power Up Your Brain: The Neuroscience of Enlightenment.* New York: Hay House, 2011.

Rinpoche, Sogyal. *The Tibetan Book of Living and Dying.* New York: HarperCollins Publishers, 2002.

Ruiz, Don Miguel. *The Four Agreements: A Practical Guide to Personal Freedom.* San Rafael, CA: Amber-Allen Publishing, 1997.

Satchidananda, Sri Swami, trans. *The Yoga Sutras of Patanjali.* Secaucus, NJ: Integral Yoga Publications, 1999.

Singer, Michael. *The Untethered Soul: The Journey Beyond Yourself.* Oakland, CA: New Harbinger Publications and Noetic Books, 2007.

Swenson, David. *Ashtanga Yoga: The Practice Manual— An Illustrated Guide to Personal Practice.* Austin, TX: Ashtanga Yoga Productions, 2007.

Tolle, Eckhart. *The Power of Now.* London: Hodder & Stoughton, 2005.

Trungpa Rinpoche, Chögyam. *Meditation in Action.* Boston: Shambhala Publications, 1991.

Van der Hart, O. *Psychic Trauma: The Disintegrating Effects of Overwhelming Experience on Mind and Body.* Melbourne: University of Melbourne, 2000.

Walsch, Neale Donald. *Conversations with God: An Uncommon Dialogue.* New York: G. P. Putnam's Sons, 1995.

Weintraub, Amy. *Yoga for Depression: A Compassionate Guide to Relieve Suffering Through Yoga.* New York: Broadway Books, 2004.

ARTICLES AND RESEARCH PAPERS

Emerson, D., R. Sharma, S. Chaudhry, and J. Turner. "Trauma-Sensitive Yoga: Principles, Practice, and Research." *International Journal of Yoga Therapy* 19 (2009): 123–37.

Miller, J. J., K. Fletcher, and J. Kabat-Zinn. "Three-year Follow-up and Clinical Implications of a Mindfulness Meditation-based Stress Reduction Intervention in the Treatment of Anxiety Disorders." *General Hospital Psychiatry* 17, no. 3 (May 1995): 192–200.

Putnam, F. W. "Stuck in the Past." *Psychiatry: Interpersonal and Biological Processes* 67, no. 3 (Fall 2004): 235–38.

Reinders, A. A., E. R. Nijenhuis, A. M. Paans, J. Korf, A. T. Willemsen, and J. A. den Boer. "One Brain, Two Selves." *NeuroImage* 20, no. 4 (December 2003): 2119–25.

OTHER GIVE BACK YOGA PUBLICATIONS

See givebackyoga.org.

Beryl Bender Birch, philosopher, world-renowned yoga teacher, and author of *Power Yoga, Beyond Power Yoga,* and *Boomer Yoga,* has been an avid student of yoga and the study of consciousness since 1971. She traveled to India in 1974 to study with her teacher, Munishree Chitrabhanu, and attend the 1974 Kumbha Mela festival in Hardwar. She traveled extensively through Himalayan mountain hamlets and spent several months observing silence while living in a tiny hut in the rural village of Manali. Her books have been translated into German, Spanish, and Italian. With degrees in philosophy and English from Syracuse University, Beryl has been teaching Classical yoga and training teachers as "spiritual revolutionaries" since the early 1980s. She began teaching yoga to people for help in recovery from trauma and PTSD right after 9/11. She pioneered the inclusion of yoga practices into standard medical treatment modalities for anxiety disorders, especially PTS, and was one of the first yoga professionals to do so. She has been on the cover of *Yoga Journal,* and has also written its asana column. *Yoga Journal* has named her as one of only seven American women in their "Innovators Shaping Yoga Today" issue. She is the director-founder of The Hard & The Soft Yoga Institute and founder of the Give Back Yoga Foundation. She lives in Great Barrington, Massachusetts, with her racing Siberian huskies, Nellie and Troy. Learn more at berylbenderbirch.com

ABOUT GIVE BACK YOGA

The Give Back Yoga Foundation is a nonprofit service organization whose mission is to support and fund certified yoga teachers in all traditions to offer the teachings of yoga to under-served and under-resourced segments of the community and inspire grassroots social change and community cooperation. Founded in 2007 by Beryl Bender Birch, Lori Klein, and Rob Schware and located in Boulder, Colorado, we believe in making yoga available—through a variety of mindfulness practices from movement to meditation—to those who might not otherwise have the opportunity to experience the transformational benefits of these powerful practices.

For references for yoga studios and teachers trained in trauma-sensitive yoga and nonprofit organizations dedicated to helping veterans, please contact The Give Back Yoga Foundation, givebackyoga.org. Our website is full of outstanding references in all parts of the country that can be helpful to you in finding a skilled yoga teacher or a support group with which to connect.

Let us all pray for healing, for strength, for an end to pain and suffering, and for goodness and peace in our lives.

awaken. transform. give back.

ABOUT SOUNDS TRUE

Sounds True is a multimedia publisher whose mission is to inspire and support personal transformation and spiritual awakening. Founded in 1985 and located in Boulder, Colorado, we work with many of the leading spiritual teachers, thinkers, healers, and visionary artists of our time. We strive with every title to preserve the essential "living wisdom" of the author or artist. It is our goal to create products that not only provide information to a reader or listener, but that also embody the quality of a wisdom transmission.

For those seeking genuine transformation, Sounds True is your trusted partner. At SoundsTrue.com you will find a wealth of free resources to support your journey, including exclusive weekly audio interviews, free downloads, interactive learning tools, and other special savings on all our titles.

To learn more, visit SoundsTrue.com/freegifts or call us toll free at 800-333-9185.

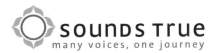

SOUNDS TRUE
many voices, one journey